D1394178

Economic Analysis for
Management and Policy

Understanding Public Health

Series editors: Nick Black and Rosalind Raine, London School of Hygiene & Tropical Medicine

Throughout the world, recognition of the importance of public health to sustainable, safe and healthy societies is growing. The achievements of public health in nineteenth-century Europe were for much of the twentieth century overshadowed by advances in personal care, in particular in hospital care. Now, with the dawning of a new century, there is increasing understanding of the inevitable limits of individual health care and of the need to complement such services with effective public health strategies. Major improvements in people's health will come from controlling communicable diseases, eradicating environmental hazards, improving people's diets and enhancing the availability and quality of effective health care. To achieve this, every country needs a cadre of knowledgeable public health practitioners with social, political and organizational skills to lead and bring about changes at international, national and local levels.

This is one of a series of 20 books that provides a foundation for those wishing to join in and contribute to the twenty-first-century regeneration of public health, helping to put the concerns and perspectives of public health at the heart of policy-making and service provision. While each book stands alone, together they provide a comprehensive account of the three main aims of public health: protecting the public from environmental hazards, improving the health of the public and ensuring high quality health services are available to all. Some of the books focus on methods, others on key topics. They have been written by staff at the London School of Hygiene & Tropical Medicine with considerable experience of teaching public health to students from low, middle and high income countries. Much of the material has been developed and tested with postgraduate students both in face-to-face teaching and through distance learning.

The books are designed for self-directed learning. Each chapter has explicit learning objectives, key terms are highlighted and the text contains many activities to enable the reader to test their own understanding of the ideas and material covered. Written in a clear and accessible style, the series will be essential reading for students taking postgraduate courses in public health and will also be of interest to public health practitioners and policy-makers.

Titles in the series

Analytical models for decision making: Colin Sanderson and Reinhold Gruen
Controlling communicable disease: Norman Noah
Economic analysis for management and policy: Stephen Jan, Lilani Kumaranayake, Jenny Roberts, Kara Hanson and Kate Archibald
Economic evaluation: Julia Fox-Rushby and John Cairns (eds)
Environmental epidemiology: Paul Wilkinson (ed)
Environment, health and sustainable development: Megan Landon
Environmental health policy: David Ball
Financial management in health services: Reinhold Gruen and Anne Howarth
Global change and health: Kelley Lee and Jeff Collin (eds)
Health care evaluation: Sarah Smith, Don Sinclair, Rosalind Raine and Barnaby Reeves
Health promotion practice: Maggie Davies, Wendy Macdowall and Chris Bonell (eds)
Health promotion theory: Maggie Davies and Wendy Macdowall (eds)
Introduction to epidemiology: Lucianne Bailey, Katerina Vardulaki, Julia Langham and Daniel Chandramohan
Introduction to health economics: David Wonderling, Reinhold Gruen and Nick Black
Issues in public health: Joceline Pomerleau and Martin McKee (eds)
Making health policy: Kent Buse, Nicholas Mays and Gill Walt
Managing health services: Nick Goodwin, Reinhold Gruen and Valerie Iles
Medical anthropology: Robert Pool and Wenzel Geissler
Principles of social research: Judith Green and John Browne (eds)
Understanding health services: Nick Black and Reinhold Gruen

Economic Analysis for Management and Policy

Stephen Jan, Lilani Kumaranayake,
Jenny Roberts, Kara Hanson and
Kate Archibald

Open University Press

Open University Press
McGraw-Hill Education
McGraw-Hill House
Shoppenhangers Road
Maidenhead
Berkshire
England
SL6 2QL

email: enquiries@openup.co.uk
world wide web: www.openup.co.uk

and Two Penn Plaza, New York, NY 10121-2289, USA

First published 2005

A catalogue record of this book is available from the British Library

ISBN 0 335 21846 6

Library of Congress Cataloging-in-Publication Data
CIP data applied for

Typeset by RefineCatch Limited, Bungay, Suffolk
Printed in Poland by OZGraf. S.A.
www.polskabook.pl

Contents

Acknowledgments

Open University Press and the London School of Hygiene and Tropical Medicine have made every effort to obtain permission from copyright holders to reproduce material in this book and to acknowledge these sources correctly. Any omissions brought to our attention will be remedied in future editions.

We would like to express our grateful thanks to the following copyright holders for granting permission to reproduce material in this book.

p. 39	Bratt JH, Weaver MA, Foreit J, deVargars T and Janowitz B, 'The impact of price changes on demand for family planning and reproductive health services in Ecuador', *Health Policy and Planning*, 3(2):285 by permission of Oxford University Press.
p. 182–3	Creese A, 'User fees: They don't reduce costs, and they increase inequity', *BMJ*, 1997, 315:202–203, reproduced with permission from the BMJ Publishing Group.
p. 47	Cullis J and Jones P, *Public choice and analytical perspectives*, 1992, McGraw-Hill. Reprinted with permission from Cullis J and Jones P.
p. 194–7	Reprinted from *Social Science and Medicine*, 40(6), Culyer AJ, 'Need: the idea won't do – but we still need it', 727–730, copyright 1997, with permission from Elsevier.
p. 20–1, 26–7	Portion of Box 7.7 (p217) from *Methods for the Economic Evaluation of Health Care Programmes 2/e* by Drummond, M.F. et al (1997). By permission of Oxford University Press.
p. 190–3	Reprinted from *Social Science and Medicine*, 53, Goddard M and Smith P, 'Equity of access to health care services: Theory and evidence from the UK', 1149–1162, copyright 2001, with permission from Elsevier.
p. 133–4	Goddard M, 'Regulation of health care markets'. *J Health Serv Res Policy* 2003; 8(4): 193–95 by permission of The Royal Society of Medicine Press.
p. 73–4	Guyatt HL, Kinnear J, Burinin M and Snow RW, 'A comparative cost analysis of insecticide-treated nets and indoor residual spraying in highland Kenya', *Health Policy and Planning*, 17(2): 144–153 by permission of Oxford University Press.
p. 137–40	Jan S, Why does economic analysis in health care not get implemented? Towards a greater understanding of the rules of the game and the costs decision making', *Applied Health Economics and Health Policy*, 2(1): 17–24 by permission of Adis International.
p. 43	Reprinted from pages 50–51 and 153, McPake B, Kumaranayake L and Normand C, *Health Economics*, Routledge, 2002.
p. 185–6	Mooney G, 'And now for vertical equity? Some concerns arising from aboriginal health in Australia', *Health Economics*, 5: 99–103, copyright 1996 John Wiley & Sons, reproduced by permission of John Wiley & Sons Limited.
p. 117–19	Nittayaramphong A and Tangcharonensathien V, 'Thailand: private health care out of control?', *Health Policy and Planning*, 1994, 9(1):31–40 by permission of Oxford University Press.

p. 108–10   Propper C and Söderlund N, 'Competition in the NHS internal market: an overview of its effects on hospital prices and costs', *Health Economics*, 7: 187–197, copyright 1998, John Wiley & Sons, reproduced by permission of John Wiley & Sons Limited.

p. 171–2   Roberts JA, 'Managing Markets', journal, *Journal of Public Health and Medicine*, 1993, 15(4): 305–310 by permission of Oxford University Press.

p. 71   Reprinted from *Social Science and Medicine*, 59, Weaver M and Deolalikar A, 'Economies of scale and scope in Vietnamese hospitals', 199–208, copyright 2004 with permission from Elsevier.

Overview of the book

As issues of resource scarcity become more explicitly acknowledged in the health sector, managers and policy makers are recognizing that economics can form a vital part of their professional toolkit. Economic analysis provides a way of thinking about problems in which the issues of resource scarcity, opportunity cost and broader social objectives such as efficiency and equity can be taken into account.

The main message of this book is that while economics can certainly play an important role in policy and management, its application is often messy. Decision making does not take place in a social and political vacuum, as tends to be portrayed in basic economic theory. Many recent developments in economic theory, and their application in the health field, help to extend or modify the basic economic models and make them more applicable to the institutional contexts of the health sector. These include the imperfect agency relationships between doctors and their patients and how these affect responses to different provider payment mechanisms, the objectives other than profit maximization that may be pursued by managers of health care organizations, and the responses of insurers and providers to information asymmetries.

Why study economic analysis?

Many of the variables that affect the outcomes of economic choices are by nature imperfectly specified and the actors involved in, or subject to, any decision do not always behave in ways that a narrow interpretation of economic theory would predict. This means that economists need to be aware of the limitations of the tools with which they work, be able to adapt to different contexts and work with peers from other disciplines. It is hoped that this book will give you a flavour of how this may be done. An example of this is the analysis of regulation and contracting in the health sector – two topics that you may not immediately view as concerns for economists but which have, in recent years, benefited from major insights from them.

Structure of the book

The book is aimed primarily at those with a grasp and knowledge of the basics of health economics: public health practitioners, managers, policy makers and clinicians who may wish to develop a critical appreciation of how economic analysis can be an aid in their decision making.

The emphasis is on building on your understanding of basic concepts so as to develop an appreciation of how they can be applied in policy making and management.

Each chapter includes:

- an overview
- learning objectives
- a list of key terms
- a range of activities
- feedback on those activities
- a summary.

The book consists of five sections:

Key economic concepts.
Chapter 1 discusses some of the key concepts underlying the use of economics for management and planning and in particular the basis on which economic theory provides rules for social decision making. Importantly, some of the assumptions and value judgements that underlie these are examined.

Although not a key focus of this book, economic evaluation will be covered because of its role as a management and decision making tool. Chapter 2 provides a basic outline of how it is carried out and the context in which it is applied. It reviews the basics of economic evaluation, outlines some of the methodological issues that are currently being debated and discusses the use of economic evaluation in priority setting.

Demand, production and costs.
Chapters 3 and 4 examine the behaviour of individuals as consumers of health care and the issues associated with viewing such behaviour as a function of demand (as opposed to need). The approach begins with first principles, examining the formulation of demand functions through indifference curves, and extends to the analysis of public goods and the theory of clubs.

You will then consider the decisions faced by providers of health care by highlighting the methods used to examine production (Chapter 5) and cost (Chapter 6), including the role of production and cost function analysis in determining the efficiency of health care provision.

Markets, market failure and regulation.
Chapters 7–10 bring together the issues of demand and supply to examine the role of markets and competition in health care. These issues have been brought to prominence in the discussion of health sector reforms all around the world. In most countries there is some private health care. The analyses of the markets in which they operate provide an understanding of why certain social objectives such as efficiency may or may not be met.

In Chapters 11 and 12 you move on from the issue of market failure to examine critically the role of government in the health sector. Such a perspective enables an appraisal of the role of regulation and, in particular, the problems of both identifying what is the public interest and then analysing the extent to which it is promoted through certain regulatory regimes.

Contracts and agency.
Chapters 13 and 14 consider the nature of contracts in the health sector from an economic perspective. This entails consideration of issues such as the motives of the contracting parties, the nature of their relationship, the allocation of risk and transaction costs.

Chapters 15 and 16 examine the application of the concept of agency to how health sector policy makers make decisions in the face of various incentives and conventions governing their behaviour. These concerns have significant implications for how one examines the role of government within both the economy and the health sector.

Equity in health care.
The aim of the last two chapters is to clarify the concept of equity and examine its application to health care. They investigate some of the ethical foundations underlying this concept and the various means through which it has been operationalized in health policy such as through resource allocation formulae and in the debate over user charges.

Acknowledgements

The authors thank Pauline Allen who helped develop the original lectures and teaching material at the London School of Hygiene and Tropical Medicine on which Chapters 13 and 14 were based, Professor Alastair Gray of the University of Oxford for reviewing the book, and Deirdre Byrne (series manager) for help and support.

SECTION 1

Key economic concepts

Introduction to welfare economics

Overview

The use of economic analysis in priority setting, and in particular economic evaluation, is often the first point of contact that health service managers have with economics. This is not surprising. Cost–benefit comparisons and/or cost-effectiveness are increasingly being viewed in the health sector as important criteria in decisions about the allocation of resources, and thus in the formulation of policy. In this introductory chapter, you will be taking a step back from this to examine some of the basic concepts that underlie the use of these forms of economic analysis. This will entail a brief excursion into welfare economic theory (and its historical development) to investigate the conceptual building blocks of economic evaluation. In doing so, you will uncover some of its key assumptions and value judgements and, as a consequence, some of its limitations. It will provide you with a better appreciation of why economic evaluation is carried out and also better equip you to appraise critically its use as a decision making tool. This is a necessary prelude to the following chapters and builds upon your knowledge of basic health economics concepts.

Learning objectives

After completing this chapter you should be able to:

- distinguish between welfare or normative economics and positive economics
- understand Pareto efficiency, the assumption that underlies it and the propositions that are derived from it
- appreciate some of the value judgements and assumptions that are involved in the use of economic analysis
- understand some of the alternative approaches within health economics – in particular, extra-welfarism.

Key terms

Allocative (economic, Pareto, social) efficiency A situation in which it is not possible to improve the welfare of one person in an economy without making someone else worse off.

Cardinal utility When the utility of individuals can be measured numerically and thus a score of, say, 2 represents twice the value of a score of 1. Cardinality is an important requirement for the aggregation of individual utilities.

Consequentialism The notion that it is only the end states that matter – in other words, the ends will justify the means. Utilitarianism, with its emphasis on individual utility, is generally seen as consequentialist.

Extra-welfarism An alternative to utilitarianism in which an objective other than utility is posed as a social goal, often defined in terms of health gain or health-related utility.

Interpersonal comparisons of utility Comparisons of measures of utility across individuals, that is, involving judgements of whether individual A gains more (or less) utility than person B from the consumption of a good.

Maximand (objective function) A particular variable whose maximization is seen to be a relevant social goal. For instance, utilitarians pose utility as the maximand, while extra-welfarists might pose health gain.

Normative economics Economic statements that prescribe how things should be.

Ordinal utility Accepts that utility states can only be ranked as opposed to being measured cardinally.

Positive economics Economic statements that describe how things are.

Potential Pareto improvement (Kaldor–Hicks principle) The basis for cost–benefit analysis. It stipulates that a reallocation of resources which makes someone better off and someone worse off represents an improvement only as long as those who gain could *potentially* compensate those who lose.

Rationality A key assumption of the utilitarian framework. It sees individuals as being motivated solely by self-interested utility maximization.

Utilitarianism (welfarism) Based on the notion that society's interests are best served through the maximization of individual utilities.

Welfare economics The branch of economic theory that addresses normative questions.

Normative and positive economics

Economic analysis has two distinct strands. Sen (1987) describes these as the 'ethical' and the 'engineering' traditions. The ethics-based tradition goes back to Aristotle who related the subject of economics to 'human ends'. The end was the 'good of man', and while it was worthwhile to achieve an end for the good of one man it was 'finer and more god-like to attain it for the nation or the city-states'. The other approach stems from a more technique-oriented analysis of statecraft, an accounting framework, sometimes referred to as 'political arithmetic'.

The difference between the two traditions finds its present-day expression in the distinction between *normative* and *positive economics*, respectively. These are distinguished by Lipsey and Chrystal (1995):

Positive statements concern what is, was or will be; they assert alleged facts about the universe in which we live. Normative statements concern what ought to be; they depend on our value judgements about what is good or bad. As such they are inextricably bound up with our philosophical, cultural and religious positions.

Positive economics

Positive economics attempts both to describe the way the world is and to predict the consequences of an action on other variables. For example, one type of question it might address is: 'What will be the effect of a tax on cigarettes on the quantity demanded?' It could be argued that addressing this is a 'technical' exercise involving simply an analysis of the relationship between demand and price. However, the process of arriving at such questions involves crucial normative judgements as to what is to be studied and how it is studied. In this respect, the distinction in practice between normative and positive is not always clear-cut.

Normative economics

Normative or welfare economics is generally seen to go much further than positive economics, attempting to prescribe directly what should happen. Because of this, it is often fraught with difficult moral and ethical issues that are, in many instances, not explicitly addressed. The branch of conventional economic theory that examines normative concerns is welfare economics. An understanding of welfare economics is important in not simply formulating recommendations for policy makers but also unpacking the assumptions and value judgements associated with both existing policy and the various options that may be put forward. Garber *et al.* (1996) state:

> Welfare economics is concerned with the means by which we can assess the desirability – from a societal point of view – of alternative allocations of resources. The central problem of welfare economics has been described by Arrow as 'achieving a social maximum derived from individual desires'.

Welfare economics has a large range of applications; it can provide a theoretical foundation for questions such as the following:

- What are the aims of social policies, for example the aims of health financing systems?
- By which methods are those aims best achieved? (This includes the policies and tools used by the welfare state: benefits in cash and kind, social health insurance, redistributional policies improving housing, education, health and social welfare.)
- How should the economy be run: in a market system, central planning, a mixed economy, or in a 'third way' as put forward by governments in Europe at the end of the 1990s?

Such issues are inevitably tied in to a wider policy debate in which there are roles for factors such as politics, culture, social values and self-interest. As a consequence there are numerous perspectives from which such questions can be examined. The appeal of welfare economics as a framework for addressing these questions can, in part, be judged on the basis of its general assumptions and value judgements.

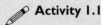

Activity 1.1

1 List five normative and five positive issues that might be of interest in the health sector.
2 What can welfare economics contribute to cost-effectiveness analysis?

Feedback

1 Your answers should be along the same broad lines as the definitions quoted above: positive economics is concerned solely with description and predicting the consequences of an action, whereas normative or welfare economics is concerned with what should happen from a societal viewpoint.

2 Cost-effectiveness analysis provides a framework for decisions to be taken from a societal perspective by comparing the costs of a programme with its effectiveness. This allows a decision maker, in principle, to allocate resources to those programmes that maximize social benefit (here defined in terms of health gain) for given resources. It represents a normative rather than a descriptive tool in aiding decision making in health systems.

Welfare economics and utilitarianism

Welfare economics is about distinguishing between different courses of action in terms of their net social value (i.e. social welfare). It is underpinned by the notion that this is achieved through maximizing utility, or achieving 'the greatest good for the greatest number'. Jeremy Bentham (1748–1832), a nineteenth-century exponent of an early form of *utilitarianism*, described the 'greatest happiness principle' in terms of the happiness of the community, with utility being maximized when 'the tendency it has to augment the happiness of the community is greater than any it has to diminish it' (Bentham 1996).

The concept of utility, as interpreted in conventional welfare economic theory, is based on the satisfaction of individual preferences. In other words, the social value of a good or service is determined by how much an individual derives satisfaction from its consumption. Key to this is the assumption that individuals know best in terms of their own well-being (in other words, they would, given a certain budget and with complete freedom of choice, consume goods that maximize their utility, i.e. they are 'rational') and that the maximization of these consumer utilities is then what is best for society (all else being equal, social welfare is increased by the greater the level of consumption and consumer choice). Furthermore, it is the end state that matters rather than the process involved in achieving it, that is, utility is *consequentialist* in nature.

Many, but by no means all, economists subscribe to utilitarianism. Furthermore, not all utilitarians subscribe to market-oriented public policy. The pro-market utilitarians point to the differences between people in their capacity for enjoyment and believe that these differences provide the basis for incentives that drive markets and thus ensure greater production and so (because of the materialistic biases) greater total utility for everyone.

Anti-market utilitarians point to the failure of the market to achieve such a social optimum because it does not take into account all aspects of costs and benefits to society. They might therefore argue for interventions (often in the form of government regulation) to ensure that such costs and benefits are incorporated into policy decisions to ensure that societal utility is maximized.

Maximization theory/Allocative (Pareto) efficiency

Classical forms of utilitarianism simply view social welfare as the sum of individual utilities (what is often referred to as the 'Benthamite social welfare function'). This construct can cause problems as it requires the aggregation of utilities. It requires not only the measurement of utility on a cardinal scale but then also, importantly, interpersonal comparisons of these. This is significant since adding the utility for two individuals in order to derive a Benthamite social welfare function entails the condition that a score of, say, 2 for person A is the same as a score of 2 for person B. Is this type of comparison possible? This is a matter of debate.

The foundation of modern welfare economics is attributed to Pareto (1848–1923), an Italian economist and sociologist, who circumvented the problem of measuring and comparing individual utilities by developing a different criterion for welfare, the Pareto-optimal criterion: an increase in welfare can only be assumed if by the change under consideration at least one person is made better off without any other person becoming worse off.

In modern welfare economics there is still an ongoing debate on the possibility of interpersonal comparisons of utility. Robbins (1932) took up the old argument and denied that it was possible to compare individuals' utility and thus argued that judgements about comparative welfare positions were impossible. Sen (1987) subsequently challenged this position, affirming that it is in many circumstances possible to compare the welfare of individuals.

Debates about the impossibility of making comparisons of individual utilities lead to the replacement of additive or *cardinal utility* requirements with the criterion that merely requires that individuals' positions can be compared to their own former positions – *ordinal utility*.

If interpersonal comparisons of utility are impossible, but nevertheless utility is regarded as the only thing of intrinsic value, then *Pareto optimality* provides the opportunity to rescue some policy content for welfare economics. Sen regards it as the '. . . natural surviving criterion, since it carries the utilitarian logic as far as possible without actually making any interpersonal comparisons of utility'. Pareto efficiency, demanding only that no one is made worse off by a change, is there-fore one way to enable judgements about different policies. It is consistent with the idea of mutual benefit and can be seen to underlie the notion of a 'free market'.

An argument for free markets is that they generally entail voluntary exchange. The implication is that parties therefore do not enter into such transactions unless it will make them better off. The next activity explores possible problems with this.

Activity 1.2

Low income countries are sometimes viewed by multinational firms as a source of cheap labour. In some of these settings, this had led to the emergence of what has been referred to as 'sweatshop' labour. If the individuals involved in carrying out such work are not being coerced and choose to work under such conditions, can such practices be seen as Pareto-efficient and thus justified on that basis?

Feedback

A utilitarian perspective would rely on the assumption that individuals maximize utility on the basis of good information and free choice. As it is likely that working in a sweatshop is preferable to the limited alternatives available to such individuals, those who choose such work could in this respect be viewed as utility maximizers (and thus such arrangements are Pareto-efficient).

Alternatively, it could be argued that the need for subsistence takes away individuals' capacity to choose in such instances. Critics of the utilitarian viewpoint would highlight the unequal power relations and argue that the exploitation of individuals somehow offends a broader notion of the social good. Mooney (1998) has suggested an alternative communitarian perspective and the way in which it would address concerns for the most disadvantaged.

Arrow's impossibility theorem

Arrow's (1951) impossibility theorem has had a profound impact on the way in which economists and political scientists have examined the issue of social choice – in particular, its role within a utilitarian framework. The theorem demonstrates mathematically that it is not possible to formulate a collective decision rule to derive social preferences from individual preferences and at the same time be consistent with a set of conditions that, on the face of it, seem highly innocuous. These conditions are as follows:

- *Completeness.* This simply states that in a social choice between A and B, preferences are complete if there is some preference existing which could either be for A over B, B over A, or indifference.
- *Transitivity.* If A is preferred to B and B to C, then A must be preferred to C to satisfy transitivity.
- *Non-dictatorship.* Social preferences are determined by more than one person.
- *Unanimity.* If everyone prefers A to B then the unanimity condition dictates that, socially, A is preferred to B.
- *Independence of irrelevant alternatives.* The preference for A over B is independent of preferences for other alternatives, say, C over D.

Given that most people would consider these conditions highly acceptable, the impossibility theorem suggests that any collective decision rule, such as majority voting, which seeks to come up with a social preference from individuals is thus bound to be imperfect.

Scope and usefulness of the Pareto principle

After this criticism of the utilitarian approach you may ask yourself whether Pareto efficiency is a useful measure of welfare. Very few policy changes make no one worse off. In virtually all cases there will be some losers from a proposal. Does this imply that we reject these each time? If so, very little would be achieved.

How, then, do we make judgements about the social desirability of a project if there are some winners and some losers, that is to say, how do we compare the losses sustained by one group and the gains by the other and make a judgement as to whether society on the whole is better off? Implicitly this requires some form of interpersonal comparison of utility. It means assessing whether my utility gain is greater than your utility loss. The problem with this is that economics is not really properly equipped to do this. (As mentioned earlier, while it can usually say whether my utility has increased from one period of time to another, it is problematical to say whether my utility is greater or lower than someone else's.) Utility is ultimately a subjective phenomenon based on individual preference. *Interpersonal comparisons of utility* require us to make judgements about, for instance, whether my enjoyment of a night at the cinema is greater than your enjoyment of an evening in a restaurant. Even if we both rated the different levels of pleasure on a scale from 1 to 10, ultimately there is no way of ensuring that a score of, say, 8 ultimately means the same thing to me as to you!

Potential Pareto improvement (the Kaldor–Hicks compensation principle)

One way to approach this problem from an economics perspective is to measure our enjoyment on the basis of how much we would be prepared to give up for these activities. (Note that this is consistent with the notion of opportunity cost.)

Defenders of Pareto optimality thus attempted to broaden its scope through what is known as the *compensation principle* (Kaldor 1939). This principle forms the basis for cost–benefit analysis and implies that a project is socially desirable if the winners were *potentially* able to compensate the losers and still be better off than before. In practice, it means measuring whether the maximum amount which the winners, in aggregate, were willing to pay for a project exceeds the minimum that the losers were, in aggregate, prepared to accept as compensation. An example might involve a proposal to build a factory. Assume the winners are the factory owners and the losers are the residents of surrounding areas who will suffer the smoke from its chimneys. The principle of cost–benefit analysis applied here means that if the factory owners are able, from their profits, to pay each affected resident the minimum they are willing to accept in compensation for the smoke and still achieve a profit, then the project will be seen to result in net social gain and thus satisfy the cost–benefit criterion. However, here is the catch: the principle does not actually ever require the compensation to be paid. It only requires that in terms of society as a whole, if the total gains exceed the losses, regardless upon whom they fall, then the project is efficient. Distributional considerations are not deemed relevant (Reinhardt 1998). Of course a further catch here is that willingness to pay/accept valuations tends to be positively correlated with ability to pay/accept and thus income. Therefore the richer the person, generally the greater the willingness to pay/accept. In this example this would suggest that a factory located in a poorer residential area is more likely to satisfy the cost–benefit criterion than one that is located in a rich area.

Some might insist that policy should not be adopted unless the gainers do indeed compensate the losers. Does this necessarily address the problems of the compensation principle? One of the biggest problems involved in actually redistributing gains and losses is the identification of gainers and losers, and a further problem is that of measuring the extent of their losses or gains. Can you think of examples of improvements where there are gainers and losers? Were there any attempts to compensate them?

Read the following passage from Reinhardt (1998) – an amusing and very well argued critique of potential Pareto improvement. Whenever posed for the first time to a class of students, objections are invariably aimed at the distributional consequences of this principle that Reinhardt so eloquently articulates. (Typically, there is dismay at why the losers need not be compensated or what Reinhardt refers to as the 'punch-in-the-nose test'.)

> One may call it, tongue in cheek, the 'punch-in-the-nose' criterion, because it permits one literally to prove that, depending upon what compensation one might sincerely offer *ex ante* to someone whom one would like to punch in the nose (but who would not actually have to be compensated, *ex post*, for receiving that punch in the nose), throwing that punch might be judged 'welfare enhancing' in a purely Kaldorian sense, as might pumping a bullet into someone's leg or, the more realistic environmental analogue, as might be shooting carcinogenic particles into someone's lungs. In the latter case, economists might convince themselves and those who might purchase their analyses that, if the recipients of the carcinogenic pollution collectively would be *willing to pay* only, say, $1 million to stop the pollution, but it would cost $1.1 million to achieve that goal, then that environmental protection would not be 'socially desirable.' That conviction, however, does not avoid the ethical implications of such a decision, and it would not make a do-nothing policy in this instance 'socially desirable.' The matter would remain a purely political problem. Economists might apprise politicians of the relevant cost data, but they cannot solve the problem for politicians with appeal to some 'scientific' benefit–cost criterion.

After having read Reinhardt, the problems with this principle become perhaps more apparent than the rationale itself. Nonetheless, it is important not to lose sight of the underlying reasons why the potential compensation rule is invoked.

✎ Activity 1.3

Briefly discuss the justification for using the compensation principle as a social decision rule and also why, under it, compensation need not be paid.

Feedback

It is important to remember here that the objective of the compensation rule is simply to determine whether the benefits to society exceed the costs. In other words, its aim is to promote social efficiency. To argue for actual compensation, the argument goes, would be to invoke additional distributional concerns that are separate from those of efficiency and not strictly within the scope of such analyses. This does not mean that they cannot be taken into account – however, whether they are or not is a separate issue.

Extra-welfarism and health economic evaluation

It has been argued that 'extra-welfarism' provides a more appropriate normative basis for economic evaluation in health care than conventional welfare theory. It is based on Sen's concept of 'capabilities' – which defines the relevant maximand as individual capabilities (i.e. the ability to perform tasks) rather than utility. The former could be seen to be about increasing human potential, and the latter the realization of the individual's consumption possibilities (Sen 1986; Birch and Donaldson 2003).

Welfarism focuses on the objective of maximization of utility (or 'welfare') whereas extra-welfarism is about incorporating objectives either in addition to or instead of utility. In health, extra-welfarism is usually based on the proposition that health or health-related utility is the more appropriate maximand of health care. The relationship of extra-welfarism to capabilities is based on the notion that health is instrumental to an individual in achieving life goals. These objectives are built into cost-effectiveness and cost–utility analyses (Hurley 1998), although this distinction is not universally accepted (Birch and Donaldson 2003). For instance, cost-effectiveness analysis might be used to estimate cost per life saved across interventions. Using this form of evaluation thereby allows the decision maker to maximize lives saved for a given set of resources.

Activity 1.4

Identify certain variables that might be excluded under an extra-welfarist approach but relevant under welfarism – particularly in the context of evaluating health care programmes.

Feedback

Welfarism potentially allows the consumption of any good that impacts on utility to enter into consideration. For instance, in health care this might include non-health benefits such as patient reassurance, autonomy or choice. These are aspects of health care that may be of value to patients but are not strictly seen as 'health'.

Summary

You have learned about positive and normative economics, the Pareto principle, limitations of utilitarianism and the extra-welfarist framework. In the next chapter you will be revisiting the key issues of economic evaluation and developing a critical review of the techniques of economic analysis.

References

Arrow K (1951) *Social Choice and Individual Values*. London: Chapman & Hall.

Bentham J (1996) *An Introduction to the Principles of Morals and Legislation*, Burns JH and Hart HLA (eds). Oxford: Clarendon Press.

Birch S and Donaldson C (2003) Valuing the benefits and costs of health care programmes: where's the extra in extra-welfarism? *Social Science & Medicine* 56: 1121–33.

Garber AM, Weinstein MC, Torrance GW and Kamlet MS (1996) Theoretical foundations of cost-effectiveness analysis, in Gold MR (ed) *Cost Effectiveness in Health and Medicine*, pp. 25–51. New York: Oxford University Press.

Hurley J (1998) Welfarism, extra-welfarism and evaluative economic analysis in the health sector, in Barer M, Getzen T and Stoddart G (eds) *Health, Health Care and Health Economics. Perspectives on Distribution*, pp. 373–95. Chichester: Wiley.

Kaldor N (1939) Welfare propositions of economists and interpersonal comparison of utility. *Economic Journal* Sept: 549–52.

Lipsey RG and Chrystal KA (1995) *An Introduction to Positive Economics* (8th edn). New York: Oxford University Press.

Mooney G (1998) Communitarian claims as an ethical basis for allocating health care resources. *Social Science & Medicine* 47: 1171–80.

Reinhardt U (1998) Abstracting from distributional effects, this policy is efficient, in Barer M, Getzen T and Stoddart G (eds) *Health, Health Care and Health Economics. Perspectives on Distribution*, pp. 1–52. Chichester: Wiley.

Robbins L (1932) *An Essay into the Nature and Significance of Economic Science*. London: Macmillan.

Sen A (1986) *Commodities and Capabilities*. Amsterdam: North–Holland.

Sen A (1987) *On Ethics and Economics*. Oxford: Basil Blackwell.

SECTION 2

Demand, production and costs

2 Aspects of economic evaluation

Overview

Economics is the study of scarcity and choice. Given limited resources, choices have to be made about what activities are undertaken. There are two approaches to thinking about allocating resources – either through the market or through planning decisions. You saw in the previous chapter that welfare economics provides the basis for considering how different allocations of resources are socially desirable. This is relevant whether for market-based or planning choices. This chapter focuses specifically on its application in the form of economic evaluation and planning approaches within the health sector. The aim of economic evaluation is to help decision makers make the best use of limited resources. It plays a part in determining how economic resources should be combined and allocated in place of markets – for example, when programmes are funded and provided through the public sector.

Learning objectives

By the end of this chapter you should be able to:

- list the four types of economic evaluation
- outline the key methods of each approach
- summarize the strengths and weaknesses of the different approaches
- explain the key stages of planning an economic evaluation.

Key terms

Shadow pricing Prices derived from values expressed elsewhere in the economy.

Transfer payments Payments which are made between parties without any expected returns to current output or production – for example, social security payments.

What are the findings of economic evaluation used for?

Economic evaluation has a number of applications, including:

- health care policy making at central and local level – for example, prioritization in the allocation of available resources

- efficient use of health services – that is, whether we are getting the most out of the resources devoted to different activities or need to allocate differently
- clinical practice – the formulation of guidelines for clinical practice.

The following passage from the textbook by Drummond *et al.* (1997) sets out the reasons why economic evaluations are extensively used in health care.

 Economic evaluation

Those who plan, provide, receive, or pay for health services face an incessant barrage of questions such as:

- Should clinicians check the blood pressure of each adult who walks into their offices?
- Should planners launch a scoliosis screening programme in secondary schools?
- Should individuals be encouraged to request annual check-ups?
- Should local health departments free scarce nursing personnel from well baby clinics so that they can carry out home visits on lapsed hypertensives?
- Should hospital administrators purchase each and every piece of new diagnostic equipment?
- Should a new, expensive drug be listed on the formulary?

These are examples of general, recurring questions about:

- who should do what to whom?
- with what health care resources? and
- with what in relation to other health services?

The answers to these questions are most strongly influenced by our estimates of the relative merit or value of the alternative courses of action they pose. This book is concerned with the strategies and tactics whereby these estimates of relative value can be ascertained and interpreted, that is, with the evaluation of health services.

More specifically, the book focuses on one type of evaluation, sometimes referred to as *economic evaluation or efficiency evaluation* (the two terms are synonymous for our purposes). In this type of evaluation we are asking the questions:

1 Is this health procedure, service, or programme worth doing compared with other things we could do with these same resources?
2 Are we satisfied that the health care resources (required to make the procedure, service, or programme available to those who could benefit from it) should be spent in this way rather than some other way?

It is imperative to note that although economic evaluation provides important information to decision-makers, it addresses only one dimension of health care programme decisions. Economic evaluation is most useful and appropriate when preceded by three other types of evaluation, each of which addresses a different question:

1 Can it work? Does the health procedure, service, or programme do more good than harm to people who fully comply with the associated recommendations or treatments? This type of evaluation is concerned with *efficacy*.
2 Does it work? Does the procedure, service, or programme do more good than harm to those people to whom it is offered? This form of health care evaluation, which considers both the efficacy of a service and its acceptance by those to whom it is offered, is the evaluation of *effectiveness* or usefulness.

3 Is it reaching those who need it? Is the procedure, service, or programme accessible to all people who could benefit from it? Evaluation of this type is concerned with *availability*.

Activity 2.1

1 Why is economic evaluation important?
2 What two features characterize such economic analysis?

Feedback

1 Drummond *et al.* identify three factors that make economic evaluation important:

a) Resources are scarce. Economic evaluation helps to determine how the allocation of resources might be made efficiently.
b) Managers do not have access to all the information necessary to allocate resources and compare outcomes.
c) Economic evaluation's analytical approach and its role in measuring cost and consequences provide a logical and systematic basis for decision making.

2 Economic analysis measures the costs and consequences of activities. It is based on the premise of resource scarcity and that there are alternative uses for such resources. The aim is to maximize the benefit achieved from these resources. It is important to remember that findings from economic evaluations will be only one of many inputs that the decision maker needs to consider. In addition to issues of efficacy, effectiveness and availability which need to be analysed prior to an economic evaluation, concerns for equity may also come into play (see Chapters 17 and 18).

Types of economic evaulation

There are several types of economic evaluation:

* cost–benefit analysis
* cost-effectiveness analysis
* cost–utility analysis
* cost minimization.

Cost–benefit analysis

Cost–benefit analysis attempts to measure the social and private costs and benefits of a project or policy option to determine whether the rate of return for that investment is such that it is worth undertaking – for example, that resources used could not be better employed in other activities. In order to do this, it is important that:

* the costs and benefits should be expressed in money terms, allowing comparisons to be made across all sectors of the economy

- the time profiles are estimated and appropriately discounted
- biases in costs that result from inefficiency and differences that arise from differences in size or scale of the operation are assessed.

Cost-effectiveness analysis

Cost-effectiveness analysis (CEA) is undertaken in situations in which the objective is not in question. This type of analysis concentrates on achieving something as efficiently as possible or making the best use of an available budget. It is extremely useful in situations where the output is well defined, such as injections given or lives saved. Unfortunately it is often not possible to conduct studies that result in such simple outputs. The outputs may be multiple or their quality may differ. In such cases you need to find some way of measuring the various dimensions, weighting them and then aggregating them.

Cost–utility analysis

Some economists have attempted to combine different types of outputs in such a way as to enable comparisons between different health care interventions, coining the term 'cost–utility analysis' to describe this process. The best-known measure of 'utility' used in this type of analysis is the quality-adjusted life year (QALY).

Cost minimization

Cost minimization studies are exercises in finding the cheapest way of undertaking a specified task – the assumption being that outputs will not vary between options. In practice, this requires only costs to be estimated.

Steps in the design and appraisal of an economic evaluation

In the following section you will be taken through the key design and appraisal stages of an economic evaluation.

Definition of the project/product

It is often quite difficult in health care to determine what is the project or product that is to be evaluated. Is it treatment, diagnosis, advice, availability of services, reduction of anxiety, or all of these? The product or project is often circumscribed by methodological constraints – for example, only those patients at a certain threshold of disease may be included in the project. This may make good clinical and methodological sense but makes application of project findings for planning and management difficult. Another example is that often only the impact on those using the service may be considered. The value to others at risk or those who simply value the availability of the service (i.e. 'option value') will be excluded.

Consideration of external influences

Consider who is requesting the study. Interest groups, including the commissioners of research, can skew or shape the study, affecting its accuracy and usefulness.

Including all feasible options

All reasonable options, including doing nothing, should be included in the analysis as alternatives to the comparison. It is important to make sure that each of the options chosen is feasible and to avoid false options which seem to be alternatives but in practice are not. Alternatives must be reaching the same target group and producing the same outcomes. False options are ones that:

- may more appropriately be considered for subgroups or different disease categories
- are more appropriate at different stages of disease or degrees of riskiness of care or treatment (e.g. kidney dialysis or kidney transplant studies, home or hospital births)
- compare different skill groups, which may involve redefining the product – for example, although bathing by social care assistants as opposed to nurses may yield different health outcomes, such differences may not be identified in the specification of programme alternatives.

These are all options which do not apply to the entire population group being reached or producing the same outcome. Once the project is specified, you can proceed to examining the costs.

Examining costs

In order to cost a project it is necessary to identify resources used. You need to define the services involved in the production of the product or in the project. It could be a frontline service, a support service, a department or even the costs incurred by a single patient. Resources used in each of the services can then be identified, measured and costed appropriately.

When looking at costs, you need to consider both technical efficiency and opportunity costs. It is necessary to identify the 'opportunity costs' associated with the use of the resources (the value of resources in their next-best use) rather than relying on the administration-based costing methods. When looking at the resources involved, you will need to consider not only the opportunity costs of using capital and the human resources used within the health facility but also those associated with the patient, such as loss of earnings or the opportunity cost of an adult looking after a child. In addition, you need to include costs that are located in other sectors, such as social services, individuals, families or industry.

In estimating costs it is also necessary to consider the size and scale of the undertaking and the technical efficiency of the services concerned since comparing a programme that is technically inefficient (e.g. overstaffed) with one that is not may

lead to cost-effectiveness ratios that are not reflective of the situation more generally. When assessing the technical efficiency of a service, you need to assess the full
use of the resources – for example, having the facilities open for a whole session,
rather than costing one item of service, diagnosis or treatment episode. The latter
approach would fail to distribute all the costs if the unit was being underused,
which may lead to a technically inefficient result. Sometimes resources can be
shared; then there is a need to assess the costs of the shared facilities that can be
attributed to the products. A full discussion of costs is provided in Chapter 6.

Measuring benefits

In measuring benefits in cost–benefit analysis, you are attempting to ascertain the
value attached by society to a good or a service.

The first task is to find out who in society receives the benefits of the option and
how much those people and others affected would value these benefits. Health care
has benefits for those individuals directly affected, either by being protected from
infection, cured of a disease or relieved of symptoms or anxiety. Health care provision may also have indirect effects for other members of the population who may
be protected from infection, relieved of some burden (such as having to provide
informal care in the home), or deprived of some benefit, because of the incapacity
of the person who is receiving the health care. Some indirect benefits may not be
directly attributed to particular individuals. You will be returning to this notion of
externalities in later chapters.

There are three basic approaches which may be used in the measurement of
benefits:

• willingness to pay
• shadow prices
• human capital.

In adding up benefits through any of these methods, care must be taken both to
avoid 'double-counting' and to exclude payments which are merely 'transfers' from
one member of society to another and which reflect no net benefit to society.

Willingness to pay

In deriving such estimates, the analyst first needs to specify the product being
valued. What is it that we are being asked to pay for? Sometimes it is for a change
in 'risk' which affects our life chances. But 'risk' is a difficult concept not easily
understood or communicated.

Other problems arise when people are asked how much they would be willing to
pay. Sometimes if they fear they may be called upon to pay, they may understate
the true value. If they believe they will not have to pay, they may well overstate the
value.

The willingness-to-pay method tends to be positively related to the income of the
person being questioned and so distributional issues will also be introduced (as
discussed in the previous chapter).

Shadow prices

The second approach uses shadow prices. These are prices which have been established in other markets (such as the private sector or another country) or prices which have been adjusted for market distortions (e.g. adjusted for scarcity not reflected in price or monopoly influences). They can also be derived from programming models which set out to obtain the maximum output from a given set of responses. It is a technique often used in evaluations in low income countries where internal prices may not reflect resource use because of exchange controls, imperfect capital markets and so on.

There are many practical issues related to how to obtain a shadow price. McGuire *et al.* (2000) give an example:

> The process of valuing the effects of projects can involve shadow pricing or direct elicitation of individuals' willingness to pay to gain benefits or avoid costs … shadow pricing of resources consumed, or released, is both a theoretical and a practical problem. In the study of day case surgery by Russell *et al.* … the patients operated on as day cases fared no worse and had lower costs than those operated on as inpatients. Therefore the day case option was the more cost-effective. One of the effects of treating patients as day cases rather than inpatient cases was to release space within the hospital. Rather than try to value the released space by trying to apportion the joint costs, e.g. by average costs per square metre for which there would be no theoretical justification, they considered how it might realistically allow the hospital to save resources, through either closing a small ward or avoiding having to build a small ward extension. This is a better way of estimating the value of the space released than by trying to apportion joint costs, and is an example of the shadow price approach.

The form of shadow price mentioned is 'implied values'. This approach looks at the value of a good or service implied by the resources used in production. Some economists consider that these are not appropriate as they may be influenced by political processes. Others, however, see these processes as part of the democratic process and thus a legitimate reflection of society's values.

Shadow pricing at least draws attention to anomalies and causes you to question the basis of decisions. Often, in a situation where there are no prices, you can impute that individuals value a product at least as much as the costs they incur to obtain it: time costs, travel costs and so on.

Human capital

Human capital theory values people in terms of their ability to produce a stream of output which is capable of being used to purchase other goods. For instance, if a programme saves 20 years of life, the value attached to this would be the production gains from those 20 years – typically measured by wage rates.

The major criticism of this approach is that it is unlikely that the amount a person, his/her relations and friends, or society in general, would be willing to pay for health care would have any direct or consistent relationship with potential loss of earnings.

Nevertheless, the fact that earnings will not in themselves provide a good measure of value does not mean that they should be omitted from the factors taken into account in the formulation of subjective values. Individuals no doubt take into account loss of earnings associated with ill health when they decide to seek aid, and earnings play an important part in the assessment of compensation by courts of law. As far as society is concerned, if there is any residual gain in productivity from individuals' health, this investment externality should be taken into account with other factors in the computation of society's benefits.

Valuation methods for cost–utility analysis

Cost–utility analysis requires measuring quality of life on a scale from zero (representing death) to one (representing full health). The most common methods are the time trade-off and standard gamble approaches.

Time trade-off is a method to ascertain an individual's preferences between stipulated health states. Preferences are 'values that people assign to different health outcomes when uncertainty is not a condition of measurement' (Revicki and Kaplan 1993). This entails valuing a health state by comparing the amount of time an individual is prepared to live in it in relation to a certain period in full health. Respondents are asked to choose between paired comparisons, with a choice of less time in perfect health or more time in a state of worse health. The choices are varied until the respondent is indifferent between the two options. At this stage, the health-state weight is calculated by dividing the number of years of full health by the number of years of bad health.

The *standard gamble* method is used to ascertain 'numbers that represent the strength of an individual's preferences for different health outcomes under conditions of uncertainty' (Revicki and Kaplan 1993). It involves varying the hypothetical risk of being in full health for a certain period in comparison to the certainty of being in the health state in question for the same amount of time. Respondents are offered a choice of two scenarios:

1 a certain outcome of health state i for t years;
2 a gamble involving two possible outcomes: full health for t years at probability x, or immediate death at probability $1 - x$.

The probability x is varied until the respondent is indifferent between the choices. The probability at which he/she is indifferent represents the utility weight attached to the health state i.

Whether undertaking cost–benefit analysis or other types of economic evaluation, a key question for interventions which save lives is how to value human life. The following examples, taken from Drummond *et al.* (1997), describe the two methods which have been developed for the valuation of statistical life.

Wage–risk example

Suppose jobs A and B are identical except that workers in job A have higher annual fatal injury risks such that, on average, there is one more job-related death per year for every 10,000 workers in job A than in job B, and workers in job A earn $500 more per year than those in job B. The implied value of statistical life is then $5 million for workers in job B who are each willing to forgo $500 per year for a 1-in-10,000 lower annual risk . . .

Value of a statistical life: road safety contingent valuation example

Suppose that you are buying a particular make of car. You can, if you want, choose to have a new kind of safety feature fitted to the car at an extra cost. The next few questions will ask about how much extra you would be prepared to pay for some different types of safety feature. You must bear in mind how much you personally can afford.

. . . the risk of a car driver being killed in an accident is 10 in 100,000. You could choose to have a safety feature fitted to your car which would halve the risk of the car driver being killed, down to 5 in 100,000. Taking into account how much you can personally afford, what is the most that you would be prepared to pay to have this safety feature fitted to the car? (Table 2.1).

Table 2.1 Implied value of life

Hypothetical example	
Current risk of death without safety feature	= 10 in 100,000
New risk with safety feature	= 5 in 100,000
Reduction in risk (dR)	= 5 in 100,000
Maximum (e.g.) premium willing to pay (dV)	= £50
Implied value of life	= dV/dR
	= £50/(5×10^{-5})
	= £1m

Source: Drummond *et al.* (1997)

 Activity 2.2

Distinguish between the two methods in valuing a statistical life.

 Feedback

The first is based on individuals' actual behaviour (revealed preference) and the second is based on stated preferences (contingent valuation). Both the revealed preference and the contingent valuation approach can be used to value a statistical life. The former is based on wage-risk trade-offs, while the latter examines hypothetical scenarios and willingness to pay.

Discounting issues

Discounting is necessary when the benefits or costs accrue over time. People tend to value benefits more highly if they are more immediate and prefer costs to be postponed. The process of discounting allows comparison to be made between techniques or projects that have different time profiles.

The aim is to find the discount rate which reflects society's rate of time preference: the rate that society is willing to pay to give up present for future consumption. The rate chosen for public projects must also be one which allows a fair comparison between public sector and private sector rates of return, otherwise merely transferring investment from one sector to another can be seen to increase benefits. It is difficult to find a rate that satisfies both these criteria.

Cost–benefit or cost-effectiveness analysis?

There is ongoing debate about the use of cost–benefit or cost-effectiveness/utility analyses, based on the degree to which economic evaluation is founded in traditional welfare economics, as seen in Chapter 1. Welfarists try to frame methodological developments and interpretation of results within the paradigm of welfare economics. In contrast, a decision maker's approach may be a more pragmatic, trying to base recommendations on a different interpretation of societal values (Brouwer and Koopmanschap 2000). In the following passage Brouwer and Koopmanschap do not recognize cost–utility analysis as a separate category of evaluation. The authors categorize QALY studies broadly under CEA:

> The general aim and rationale of CEA is to aid decision making in health care, with the goal of maximizing health benefits from a given budget, taking a societal perspective ... Economic evaluation has come into fashion because it can provide a rationale for choosing certain programs over others, which is convenient when budget constraints do not enable policy makers to implement all possible health care interventions and programs. Taking a societal perspective means that all costs and health effects should be incorporated, regardless of who bears those costs or experiences the health effects. Although there may be a broad consensus on these general outlines of CEA in particular and economic evaluation in general, the subsequent operationalization of methods shows that different views on economic evaluations may still be encountered ...

> ... one of the key assumptions underlying the aggregation of individual results is that society's preference or utility is, perhaps, a weighted sum of individuals' preferences or utility. Also, strict application of welfarism makes it necessary to view QALYs as utility measures. However, the practice of economic evaluation involves interpersonal comparison and aggregation of these utilities in terms of QALYs, to be able to conclude on a societal level whether or not a program is worthwhile. The question of whether such use of QALYs is fully in line with welfare economics is not easily answered.

✎ Activity 2.3

What does the above extract tell you about the type of questions addressed by QALYs and their roots in welfare economics?

Feedback

The welfarist approach aims at embedding cost-effectiveness analysis into traditional welfare economics. In strict welfarist terms it is necessary to view QALYs as being utilities, although one may question whether such an approach to QALYs is appropriate.

Summary

You have learned about different economic evaluation techniques such as cost–benefit analysis, cost-effectiveness analysis, cost–utility analysis, cost minimization and option appraisal. You have also explored the different stages of design and implementation of an economic evaluation.

References

Brouwer WBF and Koopmanschap MA (2000) On the economic foundations of CEA. Ladies and gentlemen, take your positions! *Journal of Health Economics* 19: 439–59.

Drummond MF, O'Brien B, Stoddart GL and Torrance GW. (1997) *Methods for the Economic Evaluation of Health Care Programmes.* Oxford: Oxford University Press.

McGuire A, Henderson J and Mooney G. (2000) *The Economics of Health Care: An Introductory Text.* London and New York: Routledge.

Revicki DA and Kaplan RM (1993) Relationship between psychometric and utility-based approaches to the measurement of health-related quality of life. *Quality of Life Research* 2: 477–87.

3 | Derivation of demand

Overview

In the previous chapters you considered welfare economics, which provides the basis for thinking about different choices and social welfare. In Chapter 2, you considered economic evaluation, which is a tool for making choices. The major alternative to planning is using the market to allocate resources and make choices. This chapter and the next will cover one of the core elements of understanding markets, namely, the concept of demand. In this chapter you will first visit basic concepts and then go on to look at how demand curves are derived. In the next chapter you will consider alternative models of demand for health and health care, learn to define public goods and derive demand curves for public goods, and finally consider group preferences and the theory of 'clubs'.

Learning objectives

By the end of this chapter you should be able to:

- **explain the demand function for health**
- **explore why demand curves usually slope downwards**
- **outline mechanisms to influence consumer demand where the social benefit is greater than private benefit.**

Key terms

Demand function The relationship between quantity demanded and all other influencing variables.

Giffen good A good with a positively sloped demand curve – as the price falls, less is demanded.

Income effect The effect of a change in real income on quantity demanded, when relative prices are held constant.

Indifference curve A curve which shows all combinations of commodities that yield the same amount of utility to the consumer.

Marginal rate of substitution The rate at which a person will give up one unit of a particular good or service in order to get more of another good or service while deriving the same level of utility (remaining on the same indifference curve).

Substitution effect The change in quantity demanded of a good resulting from a change in the commodity's relative price, eliminating the effect of the price change on real income.

Introduction

The price system is a central concept in economic analysis. The price system facilitates exchange between those wishing to purchase goods and services and those wishing to sell them. The way in which goods are exchanged is fundamental to ensuring maximization of the value gained from available resources: that a Pareto-optimal position is achieved, such that nobody can be made better off without somebody being made worse off. In order to understand these trading arrangements you need to know something about the factors underlying demand and supply.

Demand for health care

The demand for a good is normally represented in the form of a *demand function* that specifies the relationship between the quantity demanded and the factors that affect it – usually price, income, relative prices (of complementary and substitute goods) and tastes. The normal representation, as shown in the demand curve, is of a relationship between price (P) and quantity (Q) when all other factors are held constant. If any of the underlying factors such as income (Y), prices of complementary goods (P_c), prices of substitutes (P_s) or consumer preferences (tastes) (T) change, the demand curve will shift. Quantity demanded is therefore said to be a function of these factors:

Demand $= f(P, Y, P_c, P_s, T)$.

The demand curve (Figure 3.1) shows the negative relationship between price and quantity demanded, holding all other things equal; that is, as the price of the good increases, the quantity demanded decreases. Each point on the curve corresponds to the quantity demanded for a different price. The response in the quantity demanded to a change in price is referred to as the price elasticity. Elasticity can

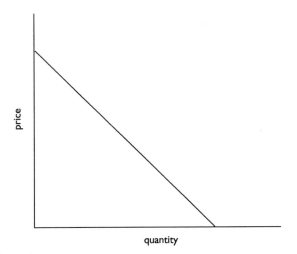

Figure 3.1 Demand curve

also be estimated for changes in income (income elasticity) and for changes in the price of other goods (cross-elasticity).

Demand curves usually slope downwards, reflecting the fact that for normal goods more is bought as price falls (see Figure 3.1). Now you will consider how you might demonstrate the downward-sloping demand curve.

Derivation of demand: indifference curve approach

The starting point for this approach is the assumption that consumers will seek to maximize their utility: they prefer more to less and are consistent in such choices. It is also assumed that consumers are able to compare different combinations of goods so that they are able to judge what combinations will yield similar utility and leave them as well off as before. These trade-offs can be represented by indifference curves.

These can be considered in the same way as contour lines connecting up positions of equal value on a 'utility mountain'. Along each curve consumer utility is constant. Because consumers always prefer more to less, any point on a higher indifference curve is preferred. As shown in Figure 3.2, indifference curves are convex to the origin. Otherwise a consumer would have more of both goods and be better off as they moved along an indifference curve. Indifference curves are not expected to cross, as this would demonstrate inconsistency – a person having once preferred A to B is expected to continue to prefer A to B when they are both available.

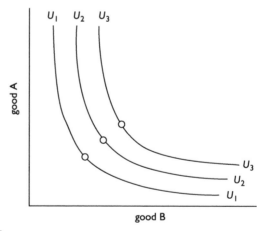

Figure 3.2 Indifference curve

Indifference curves for goods that are perfect substitutes will be straight lines as in Figure 3.3.

Indifference curves for goods that are perfectly complementary are L-shaped, as in Figure 3.4. In this figure you see that the corner point provides the combination in which the two goods must be used. Any additional amount of just one good does

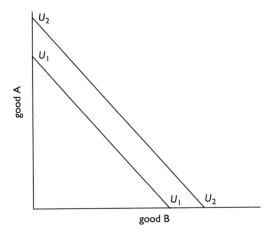

Figure 3.3 Indifference curve for goods that are perfect substitutes

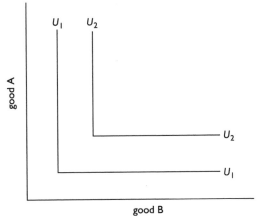

Figure 3.4 Indifference curve for goods that are complementary

not increase utility, and this is shown by the vertical and horizontal segments of the indifference curve.

Most goods do not display these characteristics but have diminishing *marginal rates of substitution* of one for the other. This implies that each curve becomes flatter as you move along it to the right. Consider two goods, sandwiches and pizzas, as a person's choice of lunch. The person may be equally happy with any combination of sandwiches and pizzas represented along the indifference curve, but as they try to substitute pizzas for sandwiches they would need to have more and more sandwiches to compensate for the loss of a pizza. The marginal rate of substitution of sandwiches for pizzas is diminishing (Figure 3.5).

You can think of purchasing health care goods, such as X-rays, in the same way. Indifference curve U_C represents the highest amount of both goods that can be purchased from a particular budget. A purchaser would prefer this curve, as it represents more of both goods. Consider briefly the marginal rate of substitution of

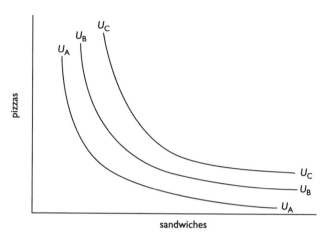

Figure 3.5 Diminishing marginal rate of substitution

X-rays for CT scans. You can assume that it is possible over some range to substitute X-rays for CT scans, but beyond a certain point you may find that the X-rays yield less utility. They would not give sufficiently accurate diagnostic information. As you try to obtain more CT scans you may find that you need to give up more and more X-rays to yield the same utility.

Economic efficiency

In order to know the position on the indifference curve that would maximize the benefits from the available resources you also need information about:

- the relative prices of the goods
- the available budget.

The *relative prices* are represented by the *slope* of the line joining up all combinations of the goods that can be purchased from a given *budget*.

At the point where the marginal rates of substitution between goods and the relative prices of goods are equal, no further improvement can be achieved. The most efficient allocation of funds between goods will have been achieved. At this point:

$$MRS_{A,B} = \frac{P_A}{P_B}.$$

Having defined the optimum, you can also find out what would happen if the price of one of the goods falls. If the assumptions hold, then you should buy more of the good that has become relatively cheaper. The impact of the change can be seen if you rotate the price line outwards to represent the reduction in price, as shown in Figure 3.6. The equilibrium has now changed.

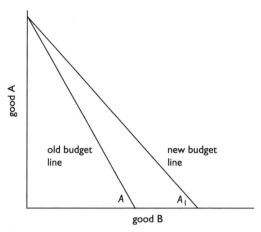

Figure 3.6 Effect of price change on budget line

Income and substitution effects

A change in price has two components: the *income effect* and the *substitution effect*. The fall in price, as well as changing the relative price of goods, increases real incomes. It is possible to separate out these two components by controlling for the income effect. If you allow the person to be as well off as before but face different relative prices, you will find that the substitution effect is positive, that is, more is purchased as price falls. From this you can deduce that the demand curve will slope downwards.

However, if the income effect is sufficiently negative to absorb the positive substitution effect, the demand will fall as prices fall. The good is said to be a *Giffen good* (named after R Giffen, an English statistician) – examples are potatoes in the Irish famine in the middle of the nineteenth century, and subsequently all staple foods. The effect may also apply to some health care goods. The increase in the price of a basic antibiotic may not directly cause less to be bought, but the increase in the price may provide an income effect – generating less real income – that can be used to buy smaller quantities of specific antibiotics for special circumstances. If the switch because of the released resources is larger than the positive income effect, then it may well cause the demand for the cheaper product to increase as its price increases. Be careful, though, to distinguish this effect from one that arises because of a change in income as discussed above.

Another reason sometimes given for a deviation from the normal rule that demand curves slope downwards is that of a 'positional good'. If some utility is derived from the price of a good *per se* because this signals its 'position' as reflecting status or reputation, then a reduction in the price of a good may also lead to a fall in demand (Hirsch 1977). Examples could include designer trainers and fashion clothes.

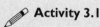
Activity 3.1

    1 What are indifference curves?
    2 Why is it impossible for indifference curves to intersect?
    3 Define the marginal rate of substitution.
    4 What are substitution and income effects?

Feedback

1 Indifference curves show all the combination of goods consumed in bundles that yield the same utility to the consumer.

2 If indifference curves intersected they would violate the assumption in price theory that people are consistent: the consistency axiom states that if a consumer prefers A to B then they will continue to prefer A to B as long as those two choices remain available.

3 The marginal rate of substitution is the quantity of A that the consumer must sacrifice to increase the quantity of B by one unit without changing total utility. A diminishing marginal rate of substitution shows that to maintain total utility, increasing quantities of one good must be sacrificed to obtain successive equal increases in the quantity of the other good.

4 The substitution effect of a price change is the adjustment of demand to the relative price change. The income effect of a price change is the adjustment of demand to the change in real income that results from the price change.

Estimating demand functions

Demand is affected by many factors as well as price. These multivariate effects cause problems in empirically estimating a demand function. If any relevant variable is excluded, the resulting coefficients relating price and quantity demanded will be biased. In addition, in health care it is often difficult to define the product – what precisely is being bought? Is it a consultation? Diagnosis? Treatment? Reassurance?

Yip *et al.* (1998) examined the determinants of patient choice of medical provider in rural China. In the early 1970s, health care in rural China was organized and financed through the Cooperative Medical System (CMS). Following economic reforms the CMS collapsed, but at the time of the study it was being promoted again. Also, with these reforms, income of rural residents grew. The study looked at factors determining the choice of care between self-treatment, treatment from village doctors, treatment from township health centres and treatment at county or higher level hospitals. Possible determinants they considered were the type of insurance coverage (CMS, Government Health Insurance (GHI) or Labour Health Insurance (LHI)), income and other socioeconomic variables. GHI and LHI require higher payments to participate in the scheme, and are open to government employees and state-owned enterprises. The following passage summarizes their study:

This study examines the factors that influence patient choice of medical provider in the three-tier health care system in rural China: village health posts, township health centres, and county (and higher level) hospitals. The model is estimated using a multinomial logit approach applied to a sample of 1877 cases of out-patient treatment from a household survey in Shunyi county of Beijing in 1993. This represents the first effort to identify and quantify the impact of individual factors on patient choice of provider in China. The results show that relative to self-pay patients, Government and Labour Health Insurance beneficiaries are more likely to use county hospitals, while patients covered by the rural Coopera-tive Medical System are more likely to use village-level facilities. In addition, high-income patients are more likely to visit county hospitals than low-income patients. The results also reveal that disease patterns have a significant impact on patient choice of provider, implying that the on-going process of health transi-tion will lead people to use the higher-quality services offered at the county hospitals.

 Activity 3.2

What is the effect of insurance coverage in this study?

 Feedback

GHI and LHI reduce the relative price of higher quality options, such as county hospitals, thus affecting choice.

There have been similar studies of factors influencing demand in high income countries. However, the literature from low income countries is much richer and illustrates some of the issues involved in the estimation procedures and the estimated elasticities with respect to prices of the good, relative prices of public and private facilities, time costs and the impact of income on elasticity measures (Gertler and van der Gaag 1990; Litvak and Bodart 1993). One of the first of these studies was by Heller (1982). Heller demonstrated some of the issues involved in estimation procedures and the estimated elasticities with respect to prices of the good, relative prices of public and private facilities, time costs and the impact of income on elasticity measures. He considered both individual and household consumption of health care, drawing the following conclusions:

- Total demand for health care was highly inelastic to cash price, income or time lost seeking treatment.
- Cross-price elasticities were significant in relation to choice between alternative sources of care.
- Patients were deterred by long travel time for treatment.
- Households did not respond immediately to morbidity.
- As household incomes increased, there was an increase in demand for private care.

Interventions using the price mechanism

You will now move from the analysis of some of the basics of demand to the examination of its role as a policy intervention. Assume, for example, that a cost–benefit study indicated that social benefit exceeded social costs but the private benefit was less than the private cost, therefore discouraging uptake (e.g. an immunization programme may prove to be cost-beneficial but for individuals who may encounter high travel costs uptake may be low). In these circumstances, how would you encourage individuals to consume?

You could *attempt to shift the demand curve*. This could involve health promotion or education to encourage individuals to consume more, or you could use subsidies. Subsidies are widely used in health care by the public sector – free at point of use is an extreme example – while free or low cost prescriptions for drugs, and welfare payments in money or in kind, are often used to subsidize child health programmes. Conversely, taxes are used extensively to change patterns of behaviour with regard to smoking.

Another mechanism that might be used to change demand is the use of *quotas* that restrict the amount supplied. In the health sector, volume contracts can act like quotas. Any intervention by quota needs to be managed carefully to be effective. Quotas set above the equilibrium point will be ineffective. Those that are below it will lead to excess demand. Some form of rationing is then required to ensure that the quota is upheld.

Finally, *price controls* can be set, but again excess demand or supply will need managing if the price control is to hold up.

Information is embodied in price

Prices of health care goods may be used as surrogates for quality – for example, publicly provided goods might be undervalued when distributed free. Three examples illustrates this:

- A tuberculosis programme in India found that by introducing a charge, returnable on completion of the treatment, they were able to increase compliance. (However, no one wished to redeem their payment.)
- In Thailand it was found that women suffering side effects from the contraceptive pill tended to cope by moving up-market and buying the more expensive brands. These women assumed that the more expensive brands were of a higher quality, even though the pills bought may have been unsuitable and therefore harmful to their health. Here price was, rightly or wrongly, seen as a sign of quality.
- An essential drug programme was hampered by fears that the drugs were inferior because they were cheaper. Marketing gives great emphasis to the positioning of price when deciding a strategy for selling a product (Kotler *et al.* 1996).

In practice, setting prices can be difficult. The following passage from Bratt *et al.* (2002) describes the dilemma that many providers often find themselves in.

Input of price changes

Consumers decide how much health care to purchase (and where to purchase it) based partly on personal financial cost, including price, travel and forgone wages. Traditionally, many developing country programmes have sought to increase consumer access to family planning and reproductive health (FP/RH) services by charging nominal or zero prices; meanwhile international donors have borne much of the cost of providing these services. But donor funding for private not-for-profit FP/RH programmes has declined in Latin America over the past decade. Agencies that once charged low fees (or no fees at all) are finding it necessary to shift a larger share of the financing burden to clients even though concerns exist that poor clients will be excluded. Higher fees also pose a risk of mass client desertion, which could result in total programme revenues actually declining over time rather than increasing. FP/RH providers need to know how changes in price can affect utilization of services and how to resolve trade-offs between generating income and serving poor clients.

This study looks at an experiment that a private not-for-profit agency in Ecuador (CEMOPLAF) undertook in its family planning clinics serving mainly working-class urban women.

CEMOPLAF managers wanted to improve cost recovery in clinics while continuing to serve their target populations. Low prices (US$6.65 for an IUD insertion and a little over US$2 for a gynaecological visit) allowed CEMOPLAF to recover only slightly more than half of the production costs. Also, a previous study of client 'ability to pay' found that CEMOPLAF prices for 1 year of IUD services (insertion plus an average of 1.4 revisits) or a course of gynaecological treatment consumed only slightly more than 1% of annual income for even the poorest clients . . . These facts suggested that CEMOPLAF could raise prices without limiting access to poor clients. But rather than increasing prices arbitrarily, programme managers wanted to understand the impact of a range of different price increases. Consequently, this study was designed to achieve two objectives: first, to measure the impact of three different price increments on clinic utilization and revenues; and second, to evaluate the impact of these price increases on access to services of low-income clients.

 Activity 3.3

Table 3.1 summarizes the impact of low and high price increases on the number of visits and change in revenue.

1 How do you interpret the elasticity estimates presented?
2 How would you characterize the trade-off between a reduction in visits and increases in revenue for the different price increases?

Table 3.1 Percentage changes in visits and revenues in the first month after a price increase, by type of service and magnitude of increase

Service	Elasticity	% change in visits	% change in revenue
Gynaecology – low increase (16%)	1.13	−18	−4
Gynaecology – high increase (42%)	0.72	−30	+7
Prenatal – low increase (15%)	0.20	−3	+13
Prenatal – high increase (42%)	0.31	−13	+34

Source: Bratt *et al.* (2002)

> 3 Based on this information, would you recommend some price increase for all clinics? What would they be?
>
> 4 Is there any other information you would have liked to have before making a recommendation on how prices should be set?

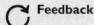 **Feedback**

1 Only the elasticity associated with the gynaecology low price increase was greater than 1. A 16% increase in price led to an 18% reduction in visits (i.e. price elastic). All other price increases were price inelastic, with the percentage reduction in visits being less than the percentage increase in price.

2 For gynaecological visits, the client loss ranged from 18% to 30%. The low price increase led to a 4% reduction in total revenue. The high price increase led to a 7% increase in revenue but 30% loss in client visits. For prenatal visits the low price increase led to a 13% increase in revenue and only a 3% loss in client visits. The high price increase for prenatal visits led to a 34% increase in revenue and a 13% loss in client visits.

3 From a revenue perspective, only the low price increase for gynaecology did not lead to an improvement. However, given the loss in client visits, you might want to only consider an increase in the cost of prenatal visits, particularly a low price increase. The difference between the gynaecology and the prenatal services may be based on the former being discretionary from the perspective of the patient.

4 Given the concerns that poor clients may be excluded, you may want to know more about just what type of clients are reducing their visits due to the price increases (is it the poor?). The study in fact found no disproportionate impact of price increase on the use of services by the poor. Following this study, the CEMOPLAF managers increased clinic prices through the system generally by 40% (Bratt et al. 2002).

Summary

In this chapter you have looked at the basic concepts of the demand function. You have extended your demand analysis to look at the effect of income and substitution, mechanisms available to alter consumer demand when private benefit is less than social benefit, and the information embodied in price signals.

References

Bratt JH, Weaver MA, Foreit J, deVargars T and Janowitz B. (2002) The impact of price changes on demand for family planning and reproductive health services in Ecuador. *Health Policy and Planning* 17(3): 281–7.

Gertler P and van der Gaag J (1990) *The Willingness to Pay for Medical Care: Evidence from Two Developing Countries*. Baltimore, MD: Johns Hopkins University Press.

Heller PS (1982) A model for the demand for medical and health services in Peninsula Malaysia. *Social Science & Medicine* 16: 267–83.

Hirsch F (1977) *Social Limits to Growth*. London: Routledge & Kegan Paul.

Kotler P, Armstrong S, Saunders J and Wong V (1996) *Principles of Marketing*, European edn. London: Prentice Hall.

Litvak J and Bodart C (1993) User fees plus quality equals improved access to health care; results of a field experiment on Cameroon. *Social Science & Medicine* 37(3): 369–83.

Yip WC, Wang H and Liu Y (1998) Determinants of patient choice of medical provider: a case study in rural China. *Health Policy and Planning* 13(3): 311–22.

4 Models of demand, public goods and aggregated demand

Overview

In this chapter you will consider different models of demand for health and health care, looking in greater depth at public goods and the derivation of demand curves for public goods. In addition, you will look at the aggregation of demand through group preferences and 'clubs' and how the different models of demand can be applied in health care.

Learning objectives

By the end of this chapter you should be able to:

- **assess the strengths and weaknesses of agency theory and the Grossman approach as alternative models of the demand for health care**
- **recognize the characteristics of public goods.**

Key terms

Agency relationships The relationship that exists between trading parties when one (the agent) works on behalf of another (the principal).

Derived demand Demand for an item not for its own sake but for use in the production of goods and services.

Human capital approach An approach that uses wages to measure the value of productivity lost through illness.

Public goods A goods or service that can be consumed simultaneously by everyone and from which no one can be excluded.

Models of demand for health care

Two models of demand for health care have been developed:

- the agency model
- the Grossman model.

Agency theory and supplier-induced demand

Agency theory is based on the premise that an agent (often a doctor) is employed to demand care on behalf of and in the best interests of the principal (patient). Perfect agency requires that the agent should be unaffected when his or her own interests conflict with those of the client. In practice such circumstances are rare. For instance, violations of the agency relationship may occur when doctors acting as agents for patients respond to financial incentives by 'inducing' demand (Evans 1974).

Agency models can also be considered to apply to the delivery of so-called 'merit goods'. A merit good is a commodity to which it is deemed all should have a right – for example, in many countries, basic education. Arguments relating to merit goods tend to revolve around access to information and the ability of people to judge their own best interests. Both arguments are hard to square with ideas about consumer sovereignty. Some have attempted to come to terms with the latter by assuming that people choose either to delegate their decisions to others or, because of their incapacities, to allow others to act for them. Such concepts have widespread application, and you will revisit this concept of agency in different contexts in later chapters.

The following passage from McPake *et al.* (2002) considers supplier-induced demand:

> Supplier-induced demand refers to a specific type of agency imperfection and implies that in order to promote her own interests, the doctor recommends care the perfect agent would not recommend. The idea therefore implies a definition of perfect agency and also the identification of motivation. Inappropriate advice motivated by imperfect information, for example, is usually not considered supplier-induced demand. Concern with supplier-induced demand can be traced to early contributions to the health economics literature, most famously 'Roemer's law': a built bed is a filled bed . . . Correlations between supply and utilisation are not difficult to establish across health services but are not in themselves evidence of causal effect. Patients may cross borders to where services are more plentiful, hospitals and doctors may choose to locate in areas where demand is high, unmet demands may be high where fewer services are provided, markets may simply find equilibria! The explanation that demand is induced where supply exceeds the level it would otherwise attain requires a stronger test . . .
>
> . . . It will not surprise you to learn that the evidence about inducement is mixed and that most reviewers of this literature conclude that supplier-induced demand is an unproven hypothesis.

Activity 4.1

1   What is supplier-induced demand?
2   Think of mechanisms used in your country to minimize this problem.

⟳ **Feedback**

1 Supplier-induced demand arises from the information asymmetry which exists in the professional relationship between the physician (the agent) and the patient (the principal). The physician is able to exert strong pressure on the patient to influence the type and quantity of treatments received. This can lead to inappropriate use of services.

2 Specific payment mechanisms to counteract supplier-induced demand are capitation and global budgets. However, in areas where you want to encourage demand, a fee-for-service (FFS) provider payment may be appropriate.

The Grossman model

Grossman (1972a, 1972b) developed a model of demand which tried to explain some of the features of health care which make it different from other commodities (such as apples or cars) which traditional economic demand theory tries to explain. The starting point for the model is that consumers want health rather than health care for itself. Health care is then a *derived demand* for health. Consumers cannot buy health from the market. Rather the consumer 'makes' health by buying goods to improve health (including health care) and by spending time improving health.

Health was seen to fulfil two functions: as a consumption good (in terms of good health being of intrinsic value to an individual and providing utility directly) and as an investment good (from which future income can be generated). Investment in health care is seen to have a direct and predictable impact on health status. Age is assumed to affect the depreciation of health stock and thus any investment is judged by the pay-off in terms of health stock and can be used to determine the point of death. Education also plays a role in this model by enhancing earning power and so making investment in health care more attractive.

Uncertainty is one of the most important limitations of the original model. The model starts by assuming certainty (e.g. the consumer knows what their investment in health care will yield in terms of health outcomes). However, one of the key aspects of health care is uncertainty about the timing of illnesses and their course, and the impact of health care. In answer to criticism of the implicit assumption of certainty, the author subsequently attempted to introduce probabilities of risk. However, uncertainty is different from risk, for which probabilities can be ascertained, although many economists feel the two can be conflated by introducing subjective probabilities. Information issues are increasingly being addressed by the advancements in information technology.

While the agency theory has some uses in understanding the demands for acute health care, the Grossman model fits very well with 'lifestyle' approaches to health promotion which imply that individuals can choose the way they live. It explicitly links health with other aspects of well-being and thus couches individuals' decisions to consume health care in terms of present and future well-being.

Activity 4.2

Compare and contrast the Grossman approach with the agency model of demand.

Feedback

Both models leave many open questions. They are, like any model, simplified representations of reality. While some refinements have been made to the Grossman model, it has some difficulties dealing with the inherent uncertainties related to health. It abstracts largely from the fact that many expenses are incurred in alleviating sickness rather than investing in health. Also consumption of health care does not automatically lead to a return in terms of illness-free days; think, for example, of expenses relating to self-limiting illnesses.

The agency model also has limitations in explaining demand, as it abstracts from the ethical codes which modify the agent's behaviour and fails to consider health-related activities for which the consumer does not use an agent. The agency model appears to be more appropriate in explaining consumption of care mediated by health care workers, whereas the Grossman model allows self-determined activities such as health promotion to be considered.

Public goods

Public goods are usually defined as having two characteristics – they are:

- non-rival in consumption
- non-excludable.

When provided, any individual is able to consume without adversely affecting consumption by anyone else. Furthermore, no one can be prevented from using them. An example might be a public beach.

In contrast, private goods assume certain property rights that enable the exclusion of other individuals. The demand curve for a private good is the horizontal summation of individual demand curves – aggregating the quantity demanded at each price. In Figure 4.1 individual A's demand is given by D_a and individual B's demand is given by D_b. You can see that at price P, the quantities q^a and q^b are demanded by each. If you look at the market, in this case the total demand is $D_a + D_b$, which is shown by the curve D_{a+b}. (This is just D_a and D_b summed horizontally.) At price p the market demand is given by q^{a+b}.

The demand curve for a public good is somewhat different. Each individual potentially has access to the same quantity (q) of the public good. The demand curve is the vertical summation of individual demand curves. In Figure 4.2, you see that the quantity provided is always q, which is the point on the market demand curve D'_{a+b} for price p. Note from the individual demand curves here that for the quantity q, both individual A and individual B would only be willing to pay a price less than p (t_a and t_b, respectively). This reflects the fundamental problem of public goods in the market.

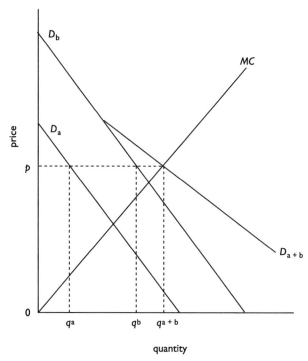

Figure 4.1 Demand curve for a private good

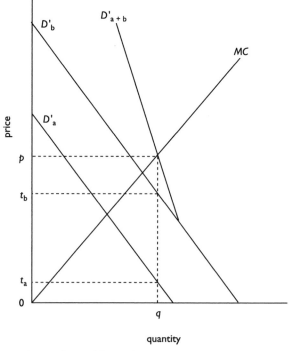

Figure 4.2 Demand curve for a public good

The following passage from Cullis and Jones (1992) contrasts public and private goods.

Public goods and private goods

A public good (sometimes referred to as a 'collective good' or a 'social good') was defined by Samuelson ... as one 'which all enjoy in common in the sense that each individual's consumption of such a good leads to no subtraction from any other individual's consumption of that good'. It was emphasized that public goods differ markedly from private goods, which 'can be parcelled out among different individuals' ... In the case then of a private good, it is possible to refer to total consumption as the sum of each individual's consumption. If X is a private good (e.g. apples, loaves of bread), and if there are two individuals A and B, then total consumption X_c is the sum of each individual's consumption:

$$X_c = X_a + X_b.$$

By contrast, from Samuelson's definition it follows that, for public goods, each individual may consume all of the good. In the case of a public good (G) the total amount consumed is the same for each individual, so that

$$G_c = G_a = G_b.$$

An example of such a good is said to be national defence in the specific sense that, if defence expenditure deters attack on a nation, then each individual resident may enjoy fully the additional security created by such expenditure ...

... One characteristic implied or, rather, described by the definition of public goods is that they are non-rival in consumption; i.e. the consumption of one individual does not reduce the benefits derived by all other individuals. ...

... The second characteristic is that consumers cannot (at less than prohibitive cost) be excluded from consumption benefits. If the good is provided, one individual cannot deny another individual consumption of the good. In the case of private goods, markets may operate such that consumption of the good may be contingent upon payment of a 'price' for it. An individual may be denied consumption of the good unless he is able to establish property rights to the good. However, with public goods, if the good has been provided by one individual he has no sanction to prohibit or restrict consumption of the good. Even if the individual has the sanction, there is no ready mechanism by which it can be enforced. The absence of such excludability almost inevitably appears to cause a problem of preference revelation for such goods. If individuals may consume a good without having to pay for it, there may be an incentive to 'keep quiet', in the hope that others will bear the cost of provision; for if they do, and the good is provided, it can be enjoyed at no personal cost. This is the strategy of a 'free rider'. Yet it will obviously fail when each individual plays the same strategy. If everyone attempts to free-ride nothing will be provided, and a free ride for anyone becomes impossible.

Activity 4.3

1   In terms of Samuelson's definition, how do public and private goods differ?
2   What are the two characteristics of public goods?
3   What are the implications of these characteristics for the aggregate demand for such goods?

Feedback

1 For private goods, total consumption is the sum of each individual's consumption: $X_c = X_a + X_b$. In contrast, any individual may consume a public good, and total consumption is the same for each individual: $G_c = G_a = G_b$.

2 The two main characteristics of public goods are that they are non-rival in consumption, so that one individual's consumption of the good does not reduce the benefit enjoyed by all other individuals, and that they are non-excludable, that is, individuals cannot be excluded from consuming them.

3 Non-rival consumption suggests that because quantity consumed is not a constraint, it is the summation of the price that each individual is willing to pay that determines demand. For private goods, optimal production will be at a point where marginal cost = price = the marginal benefit to each individual. For public goods, however, optimal production will be at a point where marginal cost is equal to the sum of the marginal benefits to individuals. The further implication of this is that individuals should be taxed according to the marginal benefit that each derives from the good. It is neither feasible nor desirable to exclude anyone from enjoying a public good. As it is not feasible, no one has any incentive to contribute voluntarily to its production: there is a free-rider problem. It is not desirable to exclude anyone from a public good because the marginal cost of the additional consumer is zero and so any exclusion would represent a non-optimal use of resources. Both characteristics provide strong support for government intervention to provide public goods.

Although various attempts have been made to determine the optimal amount of public good to produce, one of the major obstacles is the difficulty in obtaining true valuations from individuals who fear they may be charged personally for the good or service. If an individual could be persuaded to express the true value they place on a public good it would be possible not only to define an optimum level of provision but also to devise an efficient tax to finance the provision of the good.

Do pure public goods exist?

Finding a pure public good is difficult. Many goods exhaust non-rivalry as they approach capacity. Excludability can often be achieved. Many goods can better be described as 'impure public goods'. Cullis and Jones (1992) provide a useful matrix delineating public and private goods (Figure 4.3). Pure private goods are represented at position A; pure public goods at position D; and quasi-public goods at B

	Excludable	Non-excludable
Rival	A	B
Non-rival	C	D

Figure 4.3 A taxonomy of goods
Source: Cullis and Jones (1992)

and C. B is rival in consumption but non-excludable; while C represents goods that are non-rival but excludable. You will find that different types of health care may appear in each of these positions. Some goods can be in different categories in different scenarios – roads in the rush hour; accident and emergency departments after an accident. Some public health activities will approach a pure public good and some types of health care will approximate to a pure private good. Other goods will have components of private goods with spillover effects that approximate to a public good. Whatever the inherent characteristics of health care goods, it is clear that some health systems were set up in such a way that they mimic public goods. The National Health Service in the UK was perceived by its chief architect to be one that excluded no one, and no one person's care was to jeopardize that of another person (Bevan 1952).

Clubs

Goods that are non-rival but excludable can be provided on a voluntary basis in the form of consumption-sharing 'clubs'. Buchanan's theories of clubs are well developed; even the optimum size of the club and the optimum number of members for a given size of club have been defined (Buchanan 1965). Clubs are exclusively concerned with the welfare of their members, not the welfare of society. They thus raise both efficiency and equity issues. The theory of clubs can be used to explain the efficiency in the provision of non-rival goods (below congestion levels) and excludable goods by patterns of consumption-sharing arrangements. The objective of the theory is to consider optimal provision in terms of welfare of the club members. Examples of clubs in the health sector include private insurance schemes, where individuals are screened before entry. The healthiest individuals are selected to minimize expenditure uncertainties within the club.

 Activity 4.4

1   Why should the provision of public goods be paid for from taxes?
2   Using the taxonomy of goods provided by Cullis and Jones and illustrated in Figure 4.3, how would you define the properties of the following goods?

  a) primary school education
  b) public radio
  c) clean water and sanitation
  d) antenatal care within a national health service.

 Feedback

1   Payment of taxes to finance the provision of the good will benefit everyone, overcoming free-rider issues.

2 a) Primary school education is only partially non-rival in that even when it is available to all, as class sizes increase, the quality of education may fall. Although the aim may be to provide primary school education for all, some may be excluded – for example, by lack of transport in rural areas in low income countries.

b) Public radio is certainly non-rival, although it is excludable because it is only accessible to those who have access to a radio.

c) Clean water and sanitation are non-rival up to the point where a system becomes overloaded; they are excludable in the sense that they may only be available to people living in a particular area.

d) Antenatal care is non-rival to the point where the services of the antenatal care team are overstretched; once again they may be excludable in that people may not be able to travel to clinics, may not be given the necessary information about services available, and so on.

Empirical comparisons between views of health professionals and the public

How can data on demand for health services be used to inform policy makers about the right provision of services and the achievement of societal welfare? There are some pitfalls which you should be aware of when deciding whose preferences and views should be taken into account.

Attempts to discover 'community values' were made during the Oregon experiments, versions of which have also been attempted in other countries (Tengs 1996). The Oregon Medicaid rationing plan attempted to incorporate 'community values' in order to determine levels of spending on health care. The objective was to rank and then ration health services by denying Medicaid coverage to people with incomes above 50% of the poverty level. The Oregon experiments also revealed differences between views held by members of the public and health professionals in many areas. Similarly, Bowling (1993) in the UK provides a comparison between the preferences of the public and professionals and between the professionals. There were pronounced differences between public health doctors and other doctors on issues relating to preventive health measures, for example. It is interesting to contemplate whether these differences took into account differences in information, inclusion of externalities, greater rationality or different value systems. Unfortunately, in these studies, all the preferences were expressed as rankings; it would have been interesting to see how the different products would have been traded one for the other by the different groups.

Summary

You have extended your analysis of demand to look at models of demand (agency theory and the Grossman model); the characteristics of public and merit goods; the theory of clubs; and issues involved in the use of community values to define the social welfare function.

References

Bevan A (1952) *In Place of Fear*. London: Heinemann.

Bowling A (1993) Problems of public consultation on health service priorities. Exploratory research in an inner London district. *International Journal of Health Sciences* 4(2): 61–74.

Buchanan JM (1965) An economic theory of clubs. *Economica* 32: 125.

Cullis J and Jones P (1992) *Public Finance and Public Choice: Analytical Perspectives*. London: McGraw-Hill.

Evans RG (1974) Supplier-induced demand: some empirical evidence and implications, in Perlman M (ed) *The Economics of Health and Medical Care*. London: Macmillan.

Grossman M (1972a) *The Demand for Health: A Theoretical and Empirical Investigation*. New York: National Bureau of Economic Research.

Grossman M (1972b) On the concept of health capital and the demand for health. *Journal of Political Economy* 80: 223–55.

McPake B, Kumaranayake L and Normand C (2002) *Health Economics: An International Perspective*. London: Routledge.

Tengs TO (1996) An evaluation of Oregon's Medicaid rationing algorithms. *Health Economics* 5: 171–81.

The production process: concepts and assumptions

Overview

Understanding costs is one of the main tasks of economists involved in planning and management. They are less frequently concerned with how health services or activities are produced. However, understanding the production process behind these services is crucial to measuring costs and planning alternatives. You saw in Chapter 2 that cost-effectiveness requires the comparison of alternatives. Often these alternatives represent different ways of producing health services or activities. This chapter introduces the main concepts of the production process and looks at the assumptions made in their use within the theory of production. You will also learn how to apply the knowledge from this chapter to practical scenarios.

Learning objectives

By the end of this chapter you should be able to:

- **describe the use of isoquants in production functions**
- **describe a production function**
- **describe joint production, innovation, economies of scope and multiproduct firms in the production process**
- **explain the Cobb–Douglas production function often used by economists to explain relationships between production factors**
- **explain different ways economists have tried to estimate production functions.**

Key terms

Constant returns to scale Situation existing when a proportionate increase in all inputs yields an equal proportionate increase in output.

Diminishing returns to scale Situation existing when a proportionate increase in all inputs yields a less than proportionate increase in output.

Economies of scope Situation where it is possible to produce two or more different products together more cheaply than would be the case if they were produced separately.

Horizontal integration (of production) Union or merger of firms at the same stage of production.

Increasing returns to scale Situation existing when a proportionate increase in all inputs yields a more than proportionate increase in output.

> **Isoquant** A line joining up all combinations of inputs that produce the same quantity. The convex portion of the line indicates the technologically efficient combination of inputs.
>
> **Marginal rate of transformation** The slope of the production possibility curve, indicating the degree of substitutability of one input for another in the production process.
>
> **Operational (technical, productive) efficiency** Using only the minimum necessary resources to finance, purchase and deliver a particular activity or set of activities (ie avoiding waste).
>
> **Production function** The functional relationship that indicates how inputs are transformed into outputs in the most efficient way.
>
> **Vertical integration (of production)** Union or merger of firms at different stages of production.

Technical efficiency and least-cost production

Production is the process whereby inputs are transformed into outputs. Inputs range from labour (e.g. staff or personnel) materials (e.g. drugs, supplies) and capital (e.g. vehicles, buildings). A commodity may be produced in a number of ways, using different combinations of inputs.

Technical efficiency occurs when the firm produces the most output for a given level of inputs – so that if more output is to be produced we need to increase the quantity of at least one input.

Suppose that tuberculosis treatment, for example, could be provided using the combinations of inputs shown in Table 5.1. This example shows that the same amount of input for consumables could be used in either a labour-intensive (process 2 or 3) or a capital-intensive process (process 1). To know which is the least-cost process, however, you would need more information.

Table 5.1 Options for tuberculosis treatment and their outputs

	TB treatment		
	Process 1	*Process 2*	*Process 3*
Labour	2	3	4
Capital	3	2	1
Consumables	1	1	1

The above is a very simple example; in reality firms may be faced with a number of different input combinations, all of which will produce the same output. To identify the most efficient combination, economists use a number of analytical concepts that you will learn about in this and the next chapter.

A *technically efficient* process is one that uses no more resources than is necessary to produce a given output. Economics concentrates only upon technically efficient methods. Technically inefficient methods are those that use more than is required of any given input or use methods that do not produce the standard unit of output properly and therefore would not be adopted by 'rational entrepreneurs'. Sometimes you will find that people refer to something as being 'efficient but not effective' – this is nonsense, usually indicating that they do not know whether treatment is effective or not: they run into problems about what it is that is being produced. If defective or useless outputs are being produced, then clearly this is not technically efficient.

In a situation in which one productive process uses less of one factor and no more of another it is easy to establish which process is technically efficient. In other situations, such as the case of the TB programme mentioned earlier or the malaria programme in Table 5.2, it is not so clear. Both processes in Table 5.2 may be considered technically efficient within a certain range, as they do not use more resources than necessary to produce the output. To choose between the two processes, you need to have more information. You would also want to choose the cheapest way of producing outputs, which requires you to know the cost of the inputs. Chapter 6 discusses costs and how technical (or economic) efficiency is obtained.

Table 5.2 Production of malaria control

	Process 1	Process 2
Labour	2	4
Capital	3	1

This can be illustrated by connecting up all the technically efficient combinations of inputs that will produce a given output. The line that connects the combinations of inputs that produce *the same quantity* is called an *isoquant* (x). If production processes have perfectly substitutable inputs, the isoquant will be a straight line, as shown in Figure 5.1. An example of this may well be found in the delivery of some components of primary care where different grades of staff may be *substitutes* for one another.

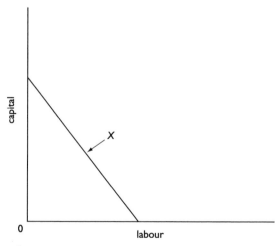

Figure 5.1 Linear isoquant

If inputs are *complements*, the technically efficient combination will be represented by a single *point* (see Figure 5.2), reflecting the fact that the output is produced with fixed proportions of inputs. All other combinations will be technically inefficient.

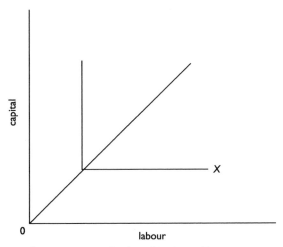

Figure 5.2 Isoquant for process using fixed combinations of inputs

Radiotherapy treatment is a good example of this type of relationship, whereby nothing can be produced at all without the machine, the electricity and the radiographer. If there are a number of processes that have these properties the isoquant will consist of straight-line segments connecting up the various options (see Figure 5.3). In Figure 5.3, four different techniques are shown which can be used to treat the patient. The leftmost ray (OP_1) shows a technique which uses more capital per unit of labour than the rightmost ray (OP_4). As you increase the amount of input for any technique, you can produce more output. In order to compare the different

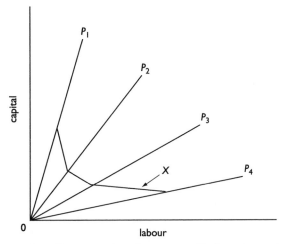

Figure 5.3 Isoquant for a discrete number of processes achieving a given output

techniques you can assess them according to the amount of output they can produce. You can also assume that you can combine different production processes
when producing output (e.g. use half of technique $0P_1$ and half of technique $0P_2$).
Thus any straight line between two techniques is feasible, as shown by the X line
connecting the different techniques. If the inputs can be traded off one with
another within limits, then the isoquant will be represented by a continuous curve
(see Figure 5.4).

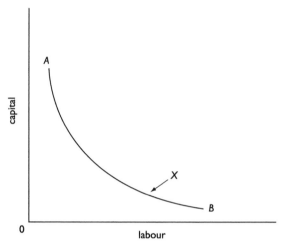

Figure 5.4 A continuous isoquant curve

While engineers and managers find the segmented isoquants more realistic,
economists tend to work with continuous isoquants. That portion of the isoquant
that is convex (concave to the origin) represents combinations that use no more
of either resource than is required to produce a given output. This defines the
technically efficient combinations.

The production function

The *production function* describes the relationship between inputs and outputs. It
shows the level of output that can be obtained from all the various possible combinations of inputs such as labour, materials and equipment, with existing technology and know-how. This relationship is often represented in a general way as

$Q = f(L, K, M)$

where Q is output, L is the amount of labour inputs, K is the amount of capital
inputs and M is the amount of material inputs.

A production function can be illustrated using maps of isoquants (where there are
only two inputs). The technically efficient production will be concentrated in the
area where the *marginal product* of each input is positive. The marginal product of
an input is the increase in output due to a one-unit increase in that input, holding
the level of all other inputs constant. The marginal product tends to decline as

more input is added, and this is described by the law of diminishing returns to a factor or input.

At other points on the isoquant map, more of both factors would be required to produce the output (see Figure 5.5). The slope of the isoquant represents the degree of substitutability of the factors of production. As the slope of the isoquant decreases, it becomes increasingly difficult to substitute one input for another:

$$Q = L^x = K^{1-x}$$

where Q is the quantity produced, L is labour input and K is capital input. You can consider how output changes by looking at the production function, for example, for a given level of capital as labour inputs are increased up to a point where no further output can be produced. Up to this point increasing returns to the variable factor would be obtained. Subsequently these would diminish and beyond a certain point no increase would occur.

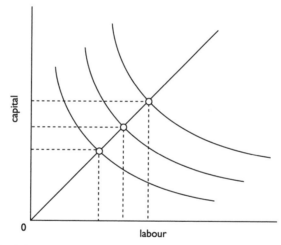

Figure 5.5 Isoquant map

The small change resulting from the substitution of one input for another is called the *marginal rate of transformation* (or the marginal rate of technical substitutions). This does not, however, provide a measure that can be compared across different processes. To take into account this problem some measure of the elasticity of transformation is needed; this will take into account the absolute as well as the relative values of the changes.

Activity 5.1

Consider a health care intervention of your choice (e.g. measles vaccination). What resources would be used for:

1 an urban area?
2 a rural area?

Feedback

> Type and amounts or inputs will vary with the setting. For example, for measles vaccination you would consider information materials, staff time specified by occupation and grade, vaccine, syringes and other consumables, refrigerators, vehicles, rooms and so on. In rural areas you would expect a different combination of inputs using more vehicles and staff time for travelling.

Returns to scale

You can also consider how output changes as the scale of the activities is changed – this means changing all inputs in the same proportion. Changes in output can be:

- in proportion to the change in inputs – *constant returns to scale*
- more than in proportion to the change in inputs – *increasing returns to scale*
- less than in proportion to the change in inputs – *decreasing returns to scale*.

Economies of scale include not only the quantity of inputs but also their prices. Market structures have important implications for economies of scale as, depending on the market structure, the prices of inputs might change as more of them are purchased. The responsiveness of production to scale effects is sometimes converted into an index of the elasticity of scale, where constant returns to scale have an index value of 1, increasing returns to scale a value greater than 1, and decreasing returns to scale a value less than 1.

The Cobb–Douglas production function

The term 'production function' describes a relationship between a specified output and its inputs. Empirically this relationship can be measured by input and output changes over time or across different units of production. Production functions can be derived for a single firm, an industry, or a nation. The actual production function can involve many different factors and some simplifications and assumptions need to be made to bring it into the form of an econometric model. These models can take different algebraic forms. A specific case is the Cobb–Douglas production function (named after two Americans, a mathematician and an economist) in which the production function is stated as:

$$Q = L^a K^b$$

where Q stands for output, L for labour, and K for capital. The parameters a and b can be estimated from empirical data.

This mathematical formulation actually reflects a number of theoretical assumptions about the relationship between inputs and outputs. First, if the parameters (a and b) sum to 1, then the production process displays constant returns to scale. Second, the equation is an exponential form. This means that if you looked at the marginal product of labour, holding capital constant, you would expect the relationship to be increasing at a decreasing rate. If you drew a graph of this relationship you would get a concave line displaying diminishing returns to a single factor.

Activity 5.2

What would you expect if $a + b$ was larger or smaller than 1?

Feedback

If $a + b > 1$, the production function will display increasing returns to scale. If $a + b < 1$, the production function will display diminishing returns to scale. Under constant returns to scale ($a + b = 1$) the parameters are equal to the shares in the total output accruing to each factor.

For analytical purposes – for example, to perform a regression analysis – the exponential function can be converted into a linear one, by taking the natural logarithm of both sides of the equation:

$\ln(Q) = a\ln(L) + b\ln(K)$.

You can use more than two inputs; in fact the multiple regression approach allows you to analyse the influence of a range of input variables on output. You will also find in the health economics literature that more sophisticated algebraic models can be used.

Joint production

Where some goods are produced jointly it may be difficult to separate out the relative contribution of the independent inputs to the different products. It is, however, important to establish whether there are economies in producing goods jointly or not. Wouters (1993) considers whether outpatient or inpatient departments should coexist. Other economists have been trying to establish whether there are any economies in the joint production of trauma and minor injury treatments.

Economies of scope are concerned with the economies that can be gained from producing goods together rather than separately – for example, producing one good may result in a by-product that could be sold separately. The measure of economies of scope can again be converted into an index so that the potential for economies of scope in different situations can be compared. Wouters (1993) analysed the production function of public and private health care facilities in Nigeria and found that economies of scope for joint production of inpatient and outpatient services were not realized. The analysis also revealed that cost-minimizing combinations of health workers were not used: in particular, too many low level staff had been employed to support doctors and nurses.

Activity 5.3

What other activities might be undertaken jointly with a children's vaccination programme?

Feedback

There are synergies to be expected if a vaccination programme is integrated with a mother–child health care programme. For example, different activities such as weighing children, health education of mothers and prenatal care can, in many instances, be combined using the same staff and facilities, thus providing economies of scope.

Measuring efficiency in primary care services

Two methods for estimating efficiency are available. A stochastic frontier analysis approach tries to estimate the production function (e.g. what is the relationship between outputs and inputs), and measures efficiency by the degree to which there may be significant differences between firms. This method takes into account real efficiency differences as well as random shocks (e.g. in the case of the specialty groups, this could be a new hospital opening which would affect all the physician practices).

A second way in which economists have tried to measure efficiency is using data envelopment analysis (DEA). DEA is a linear programming technique that estimates relationships between inputs and multiple outputs for a sample of decision making units such as hospitals or group practices (Farrell 1957; Charnes *et al.* 1978). By solving a series of linear programming problems, this non-parametric approach constructs a 'best practice frontier' that estimates the maximum possible outputs for set quantities of inputs among decision making units. Commonly used to assess efficiency, the production frontier is considered by some to be best method as it relies on the relative performance of providers within the sample rather than a predetermined absolute standard of efficiency (Valdmanis *et al.* 2004).

Rosenman and Friesner (2004) used DEA to find that solo specialty practices were more efficient than multispecialty practices regardless of whether they focused on primary care or specialty care. Strong evidence was uncovered of inefficiency of scope for groups that mixed specialty and primary care compared to practices that undertook only one type of care. The results suggest that efficiency can be improved by increasing the size of the practice as long as the type of practice remains the same.

Multiproduct firms

Some firms produce many goods within one organizational framework, and the managers face the task of establishing the efficient allocation of inputs among the various products. Hospitals can be seen as multiproduct firms – these firms will integrate and segment according to the economies of scale and scope and transaction costs (the costs of negotiating and implementing an exchange). Interesting phenomena have occurred in relation to the delivery of care in many health care systems. Some hospitals have undergone *vertical integration* by providing care in the community, while community services have *vertically integrated* to establish greater access to hospital beds. There has also been a great deal of *horizontal integration* as hospitals seek to achieve economies of scale.

Innovations

You can also consider how innovations – new ways of doing something – can affect the production process and the way in which production changes occur over time.

Distinctions have been made between innovations that are associated with the development of new products and those which involve producing the products more efficiently.

Summary

You have learned how combinations of inputs are used in a technically efficient manner and how isoquants can be mapped to illustrate the ways in which inputs are combined in the production process. The portion of the isoquant that is convex (concave to the origin) indicates the technically efficient combinations of inputs. You have also looked at the concept and effects of returns to scale and scope. A key point in the understanding of production functions for health is that they cater for substitutability between inputs. Often there is no one 'right' way to deliver a service. Rather, there are a number of technically efficient ways to organize services. The exact choice of service will depend on the price and cost.

References

Charnes A, Cooper WW and Rhodes E (1978) Measuring the efficiency of decision making units. *European Journal of Operational Research* 2(6): 429–44.

Farrell M (1957) The measurement of productive efficiency. *Journal of the Royal Statistical Society Series A* 120: 253–78.

Rosenman R and Friesner D (2004) Scope and scale inefficiencies in physician practices. *Health Economics* 13: 1091–1116.

Valdmanis V, Kumaranayake L and Lertiendumrong J (2004) Capacity in Thai public hospitals and the production of care for poor and nonpoor patients. *Health Services Research* 39: 2117–34.

Wouters A (1993) The cost and efficiency of public and private health care facilities in Ogun State, Nigeria. *Health Economics* 2(1): 32–42.

6 Costs and the cost function

Overview

Cost analysis is central to the budgeting and planning of health services. The aim of this chapter is to review the concepts of costs and cost functions, and how they are used in management. There are two approaches to the analysis of costs: the accounting approach and the econometric or statistical approach. Here, you will learn briefly about both and study some examples of such studies. You will also examine the practicalities of analysing the economic costs of a health care unit.

Learning objectives

By the end of this chapter you should be able to:

- **define and distinguish between the key concepts of costs**
- **apply cost concepts when interpreting published statistics**
- **apply cost concepts to costing the factors of production**
- **review the basic concepts underlying cost analysis**
- **understand the implications of cost analysis for the efficient production of health care**
- **examine alternative approaches to cost analysis.**

Key terms

Accounting approach An approach that uses accounting information (e.g. financial reports) as the basis for undertaking a costing exercise.

Average cost Total costs divided by quantity.

Cost function The relationship between outputs from production and total costs.

Financial (budgetary) cost The accounting cost of a good or service usually representing the original (historical) amount paid – distinct from opportunity cost.

Fixed cost A cost of production that does not vary with the level of output

Incremental unit cost The change in costs associated with an increase or decrease of input by an increment (may be several units) that makes sense managerially.

Isocost A line which shows all combinations of inputs that represent the same total cost to a firm.

Long run Time period when all factors of production can be varied.

Marginal cost The change in the total cost if one additional unit of output is produced.

Opportunity (economic) cost The value of the next best alternative forgone as a result of the decision made.

Shadow price A value which has been adjusted to reflect the opportunity cost of a good or service.

Short run Time period when at least one factor of production cannot be varied.

Statistical approach An approach in which an econometric model is built to give an idea of how total costs change in response to differences in service mix, inputs, input prices and the level of output.

Variable cost A cost of production that varies directly with the level of output.

Costs

What exactly is meant by costs? While most people would agree with the concept of cost as the 'sacrifice necessary in order to obtain a good or service', this is often associated with the monetary price of a good or service. However, economists use a broader concept of cost. The economic cost or *opportunity cost* measures the value of alternative options that are forgone in order to obtain a particular good. For example, if the resources used to build a rural health clinic could alternatively have been deployed to build a car plant, then the economic or opportunity cost of the rural health clinic is the value attached to the car plant that has to be given up.

Because there are generally two approaches to measuring cost, financial and economic, an accountant and an economist may have quite different views about the costs of a project. The following scenario provides an example of this. Suppose a firm incurs £10,000 of labour costs per year and that the firm owns machines that cost £20,000 when purchased 5 years ago. What are the current costs of production?

Accountants would include the £10,000 labour expense in the current year. They would also allow a measure of the current capital cost, which is essentially a measure of the depreciation of the capital. Thus if the machines depreciated evenly over 10 years, then the annual capital cost would be £2000 per year. The accounting or *financial cost* would be £12,000 for the current year.

An economist would also include the £10,000 labour expense. However, the capital costs would be measured in terms of the value of the machines for other uses. For example, if the machines could be rented out to other firms for £5000 per year, then the economist would use this figure as the capital cost. The total economic cost would then be £15,000. Thus the historical capital cost of £20,000 is irrelevant to the economist. It is a sunk cost and does not represent a measure of the opportunity cost of the machines (e.g. forgone rental value of the machine).

So an economist tends to measure the cost of capital as rK, where K is the number of units of capital equipment used per time period and r is the price of using a unit of capital – regardless of whether the capital is owned by the firm or rented.

If markets work according to the assumptions of perfect competition and there are no externalities present, then the money or financial price of a good or service may be a good indicator of the opportunity or economic cost. However, in the likely situation where these assumptions do not hold, there will be differences between financial and economic cost. This includes situations where:

- goods and services have been donated, so that resources do not have a money price – though they may have alternative uses which have some value
- activities have externality effects on producers or consumers – thus money prices reflect only the private costs or benefits to producers and consumers and not the social costs or benefits
- money prices are distorted by transfer payments or subsidies which are not in themselves an opportunity cost (Gilson and Mills 1995).

In these situations, a *shadow price* may be used. This involves the adjustment of financial costs to represent the economic cost. Examples are:

- including the market value of donated goods and services
- adjusting the value of inputs to represent the opportunity cost or value of the input in the best alternative use
- using parallel exchange rates to reflect the value of imported goods.

The cost function

Similarly to the production function that you met in Chapter 5, the *cost function* describes the relationship between outputs and total costs. It is defined as the minimum cost of producing a given output with given factor prices, and is written as

$TC = f(Q, r)$,

where TC is total cost, Q is output and r is factor prices. The production function, its isoquants and the elasticities of substitution are important because they have consequences for costs.

If you consider a production process involving two inputs, then you can calculate total costs as

$TC = rK + wL$,

where r is the rental price of capital and w is the wage rate of labour. This is the equation for the *isocost* or budget line. This function represents all the combinations of labour and capital which will cost the same amount.

The cost function traces out the locus in cost–output space of all the points of tangency between isoquants and the input price line. It thus identifies all of the economically efficient points (and implies technical efficiency). There is a close relationship between the production function (the maximum output, which can be produced with given inputs) and the cost function (the minimum cost of producing a given output). This is described as 'duality', which recognizes that they are just alternative ways of characterizing the same decision; this also means that the production technology can be derived from the cost function (you will return to this concept later in the chapter).

If firms are to use a least cost method of producing output, then they will want to minimize cost for a given level of output. Cost minimization means that you want to be on the lowest possible isocost curve. This occurs where the isocost curve is tangential to the isoquant. Higher isocost curves to produce the same level of output are wasteful, while lower isocost curves mean that you will not be able to attain the given level of output (see Figure 6.1).

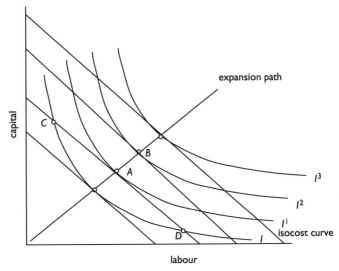

Figure 6.1 Cost minimization

This input combination is technically efficient since it minimizes the cost of producing a given level of output. If you try to define this point, you will see that this occurs when the slope of the isocost curve is equal to the slope of the isoquant curve. The slope of the isocost curve is given by the ratio of the input or factor prices. The slope of the isoquant is given by the marginal rate of technical substitution, which is equal to the ratio of the marginal products. If you assume competitive markets for inputs, then economic efficiency is given by:

$$\frac{w}{r} = MRTS = \frac{MP_L}{MP_K}.$$

Activity 6.1

Think of a surgical unit with labour and capital inputs. Explain what effect each of the following situations would have on the isoquants or isocost map and thus on the least cost method of producing a given number of operations of a particular kind:

1   an increase in operating staff salaries
2   a new surgical procedure which enables a greater number of operations to be performed at the same cost
3   a decision to perform more of this type of operation.

Feedback

1 An increase in operating staff salaries would affect the isocost map, making labour more expensive relative to capital. The effect of this can be seen in Figure 6.2. The increase in salaries has altered the slope of the isocost curve so that, for the same total cost, the unit is able to produce fewer operations, that is, it is on a lower isoquant. At the same time the effect of the relative price increase is that a more capital-intensive technique is now the least cost technique. (The unit will move from point 1 to point 2 as a result of the salary increase.)

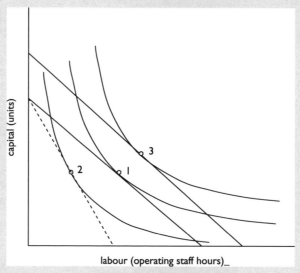

Figure 6.2 The effect of an increase in staff salaries

2 A new surgical procedure is a technical advance that will result in a shift of all the isoquant curves away from the origin, enabling a greater number of operations to be performed at the same cost or the same number of operations to be performed at a lower cost. The shape of the isoquants may be altered if the new procedure requires different relative inputs of labour and capital.

3 A decision to perform more operations would result in a shift from point 1 to point 3 in Figure 6.2, with total costs increasing.

Note that when economists are examining costs year on year, they are looking at the real rather than the nominal cost of different activities. Thus inflationary elements are separated out in the analysis.

By varying the production level and finding the respective isocost curve, you can find the minimum cost of producing each output level. This is given by the set of tangents. The line connecting the tangents is called the expansion path. (An expansion path was shown in Figure 6.1.) This contains information on the total cost and average cost of producing any output level.

The expansion path can be redrawn so as to consider it in terms of the level of output and the total cost. This gives you the firm's total cost function which measures all the costs entailed in producing a given level of output. This is graphically represented by a 'backwards' S-shaped curve. This pattern is thought to be typical of many firms in practice (see Figure 6.3). Total costs can be broken down into two groups of inputs: fixed and variable. *Fixed* costs refer to those inputs whose volume does not change regardless of the output produced (e.g. a clinic building is in place, regardless of whether 1 or 1000 patients are seen). *Variable* costs refer to the costs of those inputs that will vary according to the level of output produced (e.g. the number of syringes and needles you use depends on the number of patients immunized). In Figure 6.3, the fixed costs are constant, reflecting that these costs do not vary by output, whereas the total variable costs increase as total output increases. The total cost curve is the horizontal summation of these curves.

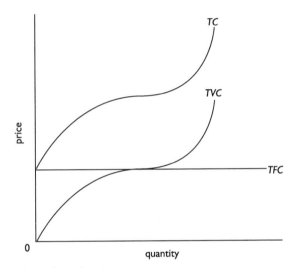

Figure 6.3 A firm's total cost function

Other measures of cost which are also used are:

- *average cost*, which is a measure of the total cost of production associated with each unit ($AC = TC/Q$);
- *marginal cost*, which measures the changes in costs associated with increasing or decreasing input by one unit (TC/Q).

In practice, without a large number of observations, it can be difficult to measure marginal cost. Thus *incremental unit costs* are measured where you examine the change in costs for several units.

The relationship between average cost and marginal cost is shown in Figure 6.4. If marginal costs are less than average costs for a given level of output, then increasing output by one unit will mean that the average cost will fall. If marginal costs are higher than average costs for a given level of output, then increasing output by one unit will mean that average costs will rise. Note that the marginal cost curve always intersects the minimum point on the average cost curve (see Figure 6.4).

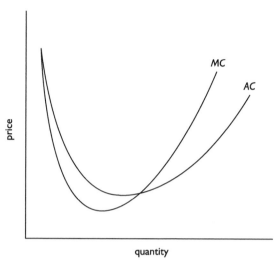

Figure 6.4 Average cost and marginal cost curves

Activity 6.2

A hospital manager is considering how many outpatient clinics can be held in a space that has become available. She gives you some data on the number of staff units that would be needed to operate different numbers of clinics:

Number of clinics (output)	Number of staff units (labour)	Total variable cost	Total fixed cost	Total cost	Average variable cost	Average total cost	Marginal cost
1	11						
2	19						
3	24						
4	32						
5	51						
6	68						
7	88						
8	119						
9	158						
10	206						

Regardless of the number of clinics, the capital costs are always fixed at $10. The cost per staff unit is $1. The manager wants you to calculate the costs.

1 Complete the above table. (Round off the numbers so you do not have any decimal places.)

2 The manager also wants to know how many clinics to run and asks you to decide. Plot the average total cost and marginal cost. Using your knowledge of economies of scale, how many clinics would you recommend on cost grounds?

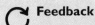

Feedback

1 Your results should be as in Table 6.1.

Table 6.1 Clinic costs

Q	L	TVC	TFC	TC	AVC	AC	MC
1	11	11	10	21	11	21	
2	19	19	10	29	10	15	8
3	24	24	10	34	8	11	5
4	32	32	10	42	8	11	8
5	51	51	10	61	10	12	19
6	68	68	10	78	11	13	17
7	88	88	10	98	13	14	20
8	119	119	10	129	15	16	31
9	158	158	10	168	18	19	39
10	206	206	10	216	21	22	48

2 Your plot should look like Figure 6.5. MC and AC intersect near the value 4 on the horizontal axis, where AC attains its minimum. This is roughly the point of constant returns to scale and where the cost per clinic is minimized.

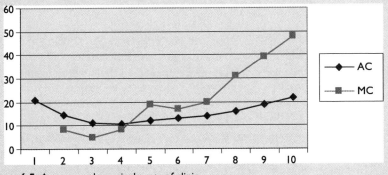

Figure 6.5 Average and marginal costs of clinic

Fixed versus variable costs

The time horizon for the analysis of costs is also important. Economists distinguish between short run and long run time periods.

- The *short run* is defined as the period in which at least one factor of production (usually capital) cannot be varied. The only way that outputs can be altered is by changing the variable (non-fixed) factors of production.
- In the *long run* all factors can be altered. Another way to view the long run is as merely a series of short runs where the firm is free to select different quantities of the fixed factor.

The traditional isoquant mapping reflects a long run perspective, since economists generally assume that any amount of the two factors can be selected. The total cost curve that you derived earlier from your isoquant mapping is a long run total cost curve. You can thus derive long run average and marginal costs.

Similarly, you can also derive average and marginal cost curves in the short run. However, you must distinguish between the average variable cost and the average fixed cost.

Although, in the short run, U-shaped curves show diminishing returns (due to the presence of a fixed input in the production process), in the long run this U shape may not necessarily be present. Rather, it depends on whether economies of scale are present.

Economies of scale

Economies of scale are present if long run average costs decrease as the level of input increases. Economies of scale may occur due to indivisibilities in the production process (e.g. you need some minimum level of inputs to produce output), or due to specialization and the division of labour (e.g. a cardiac surgeon), or because you need a large scale of production to take advantage of the machinery (e.g. an X-ray machine; see Vitaliano 1987).

Constant returns to scale occur if the long run average costs remain constant as output rises.

Diseconomies of scale are present when the long run average cost increases as output rises. Diseconomies of scale may arise because as you increase the output produced you may find that additional costs arise (e.g. overtime for nurses, or you need to rent additional space as your clinic gets overcrowded).

If you have a U-shaped long run average cost curve there is a range of output for which there are economies of scale and diseconomies of scale. From the left, the curve turns downwards to q_1 indicating economies of scale. Between q_1 and q_2 there are more or less constant returns to scale as the curve is almost horizontal. From q_2 onwards, diseconomies of scale are exhibited as the curve then bends upwards (see Figure 6.6). Remember that the discussion of economies of scale takes place only in the long run context.

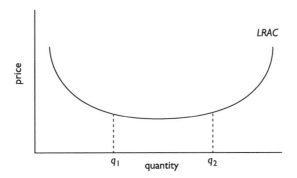

production up to point q_1 indicates economies of scale
production beyond point q_2 indicates diseconomies of scale

Figure 6.6 Long run average cost curve

Economies of scope

A related concept is that of economies of scope which you considered in the previous chapter. These are possible only in the context of a firm producing more than one type of output. Economies of scope occur when it is possible to produce jointly two or more outputs of different goods, more cheaply than they can be produced separately.

Weaver and Deolalikar (2004) undertook a study of the economies of scale and scope in Vietnamese hospitals. The following extract describes some of their findings:

> Historically, public hospitals in Vietnam were allocated primarily by administrative units rather than by a market. In a system of public hospitals that follows an administrative structure, returns to scale may depend on the category of hospital in addition to the number of beds and volume of output. Most previous research on returns to scale has focused on the number of beds and volume of output. For example, a recent review reported consistent evidence of economies of scale for hospitals with 100–200 beds, and diseconomies of scale for hospitals with 300–600 beds ... In contrast, in Vietnam the central general hospitals with a mean of 561 beds exhibited constant returns to scale, as did the central specialty hospitals with a mean of 226 beds. Provincial general hospitals with a mean of 357 beds and provincial specialty hospitals with a mean of 192 beds exhibited decreasing returns to scale. Among the smaller hospitals, district hospitals with a mean of 76 beds exhibited increasing returns to scale, whereas other ministry hospitals with a mean of 84 beds exhibited decreasing returns to scale.

They constructed an economies of scale index from their results (Table 6.2). If this is around 1, then constant returns to scale are indicated; if it is less than 1, then diseconomies of scale are present, and if it is greater than 1, then increasing returns are present.

Table 6.2 Economies of scale and scope in Vietnamese hospitals

Type of hospital	Average number of beds	Economies of scale index	Economies of scope index
District	76	1.16	0.05
Other ministry	84	0.89	0.01
Provincial specialty	192	0.58	0.18
Provincial general	357	0.20	0.61
Central specialty	226	1.05	0.05
Central general	561	1.09	0.48

Source: Weaver and Deolalikar (2004)

Activity 6.3

1 Which hospitals are scale efficient?
2 What do the results suggest about hospital management in Vietnam?
3 The economies of scope index measures whether it was more or less expensive to provide both inpatient and outpatient care. If this measure is greater than zero, it is more efficient to provide both. If the scope index is less than zero then there would not be economies of scope. What would you advise policy makers about combining inpatient and outpatient services from these data?

Feedback

1 The economies of scale index for the central general and central specialty hospitals is close to 1, indicating constant returns to scale, and so there is scale efficiency.

2 This analysis suggests that the managerial resources that were allocated by administrative unit could perhaps be more efficiently allocated. The results related to the provincial hospitals suggest that it might be worthwhile to consider how to divide these into smaller units.

3 The economies of scope indices were all greater than zero. In particular, central and provincial general hospitals showed large economies of scope relative to central speciality, district and other ministry hospitals.

Approaches to cost and efficiency analysis

There are two ways of exploring cost and efficiency issues in health: the accounting approach (also called the unit costing approach) and statistical cost analysis.

The accounting approach

This approach uses accounting information to do either a strict accounting analysis or economic costing. The data can be collected from one hospital or health centre with detailed examination of the resources via the accounts. This is the type of cost analysis that is used in economic evaluation. The cost analysis can be done from the perspective of the organization (e.g. what are the resources used in producing this service or good?) or from the perspective of a society as a whole (e.g. what are the total resources needed to perform this service?). Such studies are often called 'unit cost' studies as they yield values for average costs. People often use average variable costs as a proxy for marginal costs in these studies. These studies are often used to compare relative efficiency across activities or hospitals (Barnum and Kutzin 1993).

Although it is widely used, there are a number of shortcomings to this approach.

1 Average cost information is not sufficient to make judgements about economic efficiency. For example, if the issue is whether a service should be expanded beyond its current level, it is more important to look at the marginal cost; average cost does not tell you what is likely to happen as price or output changes. Thus the implicit assumption of an accounting cost function is that the underlying cost curve is linear and thus the marginal costs are constant. You cannot test if this assumption is correct.

2 Under ideal conditions, a study comparing average costs across hospitals would tell you which one provided the services with the greatest efficiency, but this does not include taking into account factors such as the quality of services in each facility, the case mix (composition of types of patient), and the fact that, to measure economic efficiency, the cost information would have to measure the social opportunity cost of the resources. Thus high average costs could indicate high quality, complicated patients, or low efficiency.

3 Accounting cost functions represent the cost of production at one point in time; the accounting approach cannot therefore be used to examine concepts such as economies of scale which occur over time. The accounting view of the cost function is rigid in the sense that it does not allow management to respond to changes in output prices or quantities. The accounting study only yields one point along the total cost curve.

The following passage describes a cost analysis of insecticide-treated nets and indoor residual spraying in Kenya to prevent malaria (Guyatt *et al.* 2002).

A retrospective cost analysis of the vector control activities for a 1-year period was undertaken in consultation with the Merlin team. A financial analysis (cash expenditures) was undertaken from the providers' perspective, both with and without costs recovered from the sale of nets. The average cost per net recovered was estimated at Ksh. 249.38 (from the sale of 125 nets at Ksh. 50 and 275 nets at Ksh. 340. with Ksh. 10 from these nets being retained by the group). This assumes that all payments made were recovered from the groups. The financial analysis includes the cost of the Merlin staff assigned to the office in Kisii but excludes costs for the office in Nairobi. An economic analysis was also undertaken from a societal perspective that annualized the cost of training (over 2 years), nets (over 5 years), spraying pumps (over 8 years) and megaphones (over 10 years), assuming a discount rate of 3 % . . . The economic costs also included the opportunity costs of using existing MOH staff, government civil administration staff and members of the community, and the Merlin truck to transport material from Nairobi to Kisii. The opportunity costs for using existing personnel were assessed as daily gross salaries (MOH and Administration) or the average daily income for casual labour in the rural areas (community members).

The opportunity cost of using existing pumps (MOH or community) was not assessed.

The results obtained are shown in Table 6.3.

Table 6.3 Cost per person protected of indoor residual house spraying (IRS) and insecticide-treated bednets (ITN) in the first year of operation (2000)

Cost analysis	Cost centre	Financial		Economic	
		Cost (Ksh.)	% of total costs	Cost (Ksh.)	% of total costs
IRS	Priority areas identification	0.33	0.5	0.42	0.6
	Training	1.06	1.6	0.66	1.0
	Implementation	0.79	1.2	0.79	1.1
	Project	13.70	20.4	15.54	22.6
	Insecticide (Icon)	51.28	76.3	51.29	74.7
	Total	67.16 (US$0.86)		68.70 (US$0.88)	
ITN	Bednet group identification	23.62	7.2	25.08	13.7
	Bednet group training	80.27	24.3	47.34	25.8
	Bednet group monitoring	33.75	10.2	35.25	19.2
	Project	6.02	1.8	6.02	3.3
	Nets	150.97	45.8	34.34	18.7
	Insecticide (K-Othrine)	35.25	10.7	35.28	19.3
	Total	329.88 (US$4.21)		183.31 (US$2.34)	

Source: Guyatt *et al.* (2002)

Activity 6.4

1 Considering the definition of opportunity costs given earlier, do you think the cost analysis presented by Guyatt *et al.* provides an accounting or economic approach to cost analysis? What costs do they use? What factors contribute to your conclusion?
2 What might be some reasons why economic costs differ from financial costs?
3 What can you tell about how costs might change as the number of people or households protected increase?

Feedback

1 Guyatt *et al.* present the costs of malaria prevention activities in Kenya using an accounting-type analysis. They present a typical breakdown of costs by input category. They can derive a unit or average cost per person protected by dividing the cost per treated net sold by the number of people covered by a single net.

2 Key differences between the financial and economic costs are that in the financial

analysis the net cash outlay for the net (a capital item) is assigned to the first year. In the economic costing the cost of all capital items is distributed over the life expectancy of each item. The economic costs also include the opportunity costs for existing resources such as personnel and community volunteers. Given that they have left out expatriate salaries (which constitute a large amount of the total project budget), they are most likely presenting financial costs.

3 The 'unit-cost' approach captures costs only at one moment in time or scale of activity. This type of cost analysis only allows you to extrapolate what would happen if the project were enlarged. For example, you could assume constant average costs and say that the cost of the activity would increase proportionately with the number of people protected. Alternatively, you could assume that it might cost more or less as you expand the programme. However, this unit-cost approach does not give you any guidance on the returns to scale of this project.

Statistical cost functions

Statistical or econometric analysis of cost functions allows you to get a better idea of how total costs change in response to differences in service mix, inputs, input prices and the level of output. For example, if you had an increase in the price of one factor, an accounting approach would show that total costs would rise by the increase in price and the amount of the factor that is used. However, the econometric model would allow for total costs to rise at a rate less than the price increase to allow for substitution of other factors and the decrease in the use of the factor whose price has increased.

Consider what would happen if there was an increase in the cost of doctor time. Would the unit cost of a tuberculosis care scheme in a communicable disease clinic be likely to increase, or would a substitute for the doctor be considered?

The *statistical approach* does not focus on individual units or activities; rather it looks at why costs differ. You need to have a statistical cost function to derive estimates for marginal costs, and economies of scale and scope.

Estimation of statistical cost functions requires data on a relatively large number of units. The basic methodology is that you specify a cost function that you want to estimate (e.g. you may think that it is a Cobb–Douglas specification) and then use regression techniques to estimate the parameters. Wouters (1993) estimated a statistical cost function and used this information to calculate whether there were economies of scope between inpatient and outpatient services, finding no evidence of economies of scope. Activity 6.3 about Vietnamese hospitals also involved statistical techniques in order to understand the costs.

The statistical cost function is often called a behavioural cost function since it is based on observed information. However, this actual behaviour may not be cost-minimizing. There are some key issues which emerge when actually estimating a statistical cost function (Tatchell 1983):

• how to define/measure output (e.g. is it patient days, improvement in health status?)

- the need to control for case mix and quality of services
- lack of data.

Nevertheless, there have been many statistical cost function studies in high-income countries, as you saw in the previous chapter. In the American literature, early studies of hospitals found evidence of economies of scale and an optimum size of about 250 beds. Recent contributions suggest no economies or perhaps even some diseconomies of scale. In contrast, studies on individual services, such as open heart surgery, find evidence of economies of scale. One explanation for these results is that economies of scale do occur for certain services but are offset by other services with diseconomies of scale within the hospital.

Wagstaff's (1989) review of British cost studies found one study (Gray *et al.* 1986) where there was a high degree of substitutability between capital and labour and between professional/technical staff and domestic/ancillary staff, but a fairly high degree of complementarity between medical staff and professional/technical staff.

The following is the introduction and conclusion of a paper by Simpson (1995) which discusses the impact of hospital size:

> A number of health care analysts have argued that small hospitals could deliver health care more efficiently if they were allowed to attain a larger scale through merger. Previous studies of the minimum efficient scale for hospitals, which find that hospitals continue to realize economies of scale up to 200 beds and that sub-100 bed hospitals are particularly inefficient, generally support this position. This note, however, presents some contrary evidence: Fourteen of the twenty general acute-care hospitals that have recently opened in California have fewer than 100 licensed beds, and eighteen have fewer than 200 licensed beds. . . .
>
> Previous studies of minimum efficient scale can be divided into two groups. Studies of hospital cost functions, which comprise the first group, generally suggest that hospitals continue to realize economies of scale up to 200 beds. However, there are three reasons to question whether the results of these studies can be used to determine the current minimum efficient scale. First . . . even the more careful studies have limitations that make it difficult to infer the long-run minimum efficient scale. Second, studies of hospital cost functions ignore the patient's transportation costs. Thus, while these studies can show how to minimize the cost of producing hospital services, they cannot show how to minimize the total cost of producing and delivering hospital services to patients. Third, the competitive conditions in the hospital industry during the periods examined by these studies differ substantially from current competitive conditions. For instance, hospitals are thought to have competed for physician loyalty by offering a higher quality of care during the time period examined by many of these studies. One component of this quality was excess bed capacity . . . Now that third party payers are demanding that hospitals compete on price as well as quality, minimum efficient size may be smaller because hospitals presumably maintain less excess bed capacity.

✎ Activity 6.5

Briefly, what reasons does the author give for arguing that hospitals with less than 100 beds are more efficient than previous studies suggest?

Feedback

The author argues that hospital facilities in California with less than 100 beds are more efficient than previously thought. This is because small facilities are competing with larger hospitals, which are located nearby. This may indicate that the small hospitals can compete through the level of services provided and may be more efficient for the local consumer (taking into account travel costs and so on.). The reduction in smaller facilities may not have been because of inefficiency of service provision but rather through government entry restrictions which prevent the replacement of older facilities.

There have been very few such studies in low-income countries. There is no consistent outcome regarding whether hospitals are facing returns to scale. For an economist, the two approaches (accounting and statistical cost functions) can be seen as complementary to understanding the nature of costs and production facing a health care unit.

 Activity 6.6

Test your knowledge of this chapter by closing the book and writing notes on the following:

1 opportunity cost
2 the cost function
3 the difference between an isocost and an isoquant
4 the relationship between average and marginal cost
5 what happens to the average cost curve when increasing, constant and decreasing returns to scale are present (draw a curve to represent these relationships).

 Feedback

The following are only brief answers for you to check your understanding. Your notes should be fuller than these.

1 Opportunity cost is the cost of a good or service, valued by an estimation of using the same resources in the next best alternative use.

2 The cost function is the relationship between outputs and total costs: $TC = f(Q, r)$, where Q = output and r = factor prices.

3 An isocost is a line which shows all combinations of inputs that represent the same total cost to a firm, whereas an isoquant is a line joining up all combinations of inputs that produce the same quantity.

4 If marginal costs are less than average costs for a given level of output, then increasing output by a unit will mean that the average cost will fall. If marginal costs are greater than average costs for a given level of output, then increasing output by one unit will mean that average costs will now increase. The marginal cost curve always cuts through the minimum point on the average cost curve.

5 Your long run average cost curve should be similar to that shown in Figure 6.4. Increasing returns to scale will be present where average cost is falling, constant returns to scale are constant along the (flat) lowest portion of the curve, and where average costs rise as output rises there will be diminishing returns to scale.

Summary

You have learned about the concepts of costs and the cost function and seen how the cost function can be used in conjunction with the production function to determine the least cost method of production. You went on to learn about the accounting and statistical cost function approaches used to explore cost and efficiency in health, and looked at examples of how these methods have been applied.

References

Barnum H and Kutzin J (1993) *Public Hospitals in Developing Countries: Resource Use, Cost and Financing*. Baltimore, MD: Johns Hopkins University Press.

Gilson L and Mills A (1995) Health sector reforms in sub-Saharan Africa: lessons of the last 10 years. *Health Policy* 32: 215–43.

Gray A, McGuire A and Stuart P (1986) Factor input in NHS hospitals. Discussion Paper 02/86, University of Aberdeen Health Economics Research Unit, Aberdeen.

Guyatt HL, Kinnear J, Burinin M and Snow RW (2002) A comparative cost analysis of insecticide-treated nets and indoor residual spraying in highland Kenya. *Health Policy and Planning* 17(2): 144–53.

Simpson J (1995) A note on entry by small hospitals. *Journal of Health Economics* 14: 107–13.

Tatchell M (1983) Measuring hospital output: A review of the service-mix and case-mix approaches. *Social Science & Medicine* 27(13): 871–87.

Vitaliano DF (1987) On the estimation of hospital cost functions. *Journal of Health Economics* 6: 305–18.

Wagstaff A (1989) Econometric studies in health economics. A survey of the British Literature. *Journal of Health Economics* 8: 1–51.

Weaver M and Deolalikar A (2004) Economies of scale and scope in Vietnamese hospitals. *Social Science & Medicine* 59: 199–208.

Wouters A (1993) The cost and efficiency of public and private health care facilities in Ogun State, Nigeria. *Health Economics* 2(1): 32–42.

Markets, market failure and regulation

Market analysis

Overview

In this chapter you will revise the key concepts of supply and demand in the marketplace, consider the relevance of market analysis to health care and analyse the different market structures, looking at their implications for the provision of health care.

Learning objectives

By the end of this chapter you should be able to:

- discuss the relevance of market analysis to health care
- explain the key assumptions of perfect competition
- define points of consumption and production in a perfectly competitive market
- explain why markets are unlikely to be perfectly competitive
- discuss the imperfect competition structure of oligopolies
- discuss the role of game theory in the market
- discuss the role of asymmetrical information in the marketplace.

Key terms

Contestable market A market where monopolistic behaviour is disciplined by the threat of entry into the market by other firms.

Equilibrium A state where (in the context of the market) supply is equal to demand and price is stable.

Homogeneous goods Goods which seem identical in the eyes of the consumer.

Laissez-faire Economic philosophy that relies on market mechanisms to allocate goods and services.

Marginal revenue The change in total revenue resulting from selling one more unit of output.

Market failure The failure of an unregulated market to achieve an efficient allocation of resources.

Monopoly Situation where there is only one supplier of a product.

Monopsony Situation where there is only one buyer in the market.

Normal profit The rate of return that is earned in a competitive market. It is usually incorporated in costs. If profits above normal are earned the market will attract new entrants unless there are barriers to entry.

Oligopoly A market that contains only a few firms.

Prisoners' dilemma (collective action problem) Situation where the collective interests of a group are inconsistent with the individual interests of its members. The problem with achieving the necessary cooperation among group members is that, in cooperating, each individual opens him- or herself to exploitation from the others.

Sunk costs Costs that are non-recoverable.

Supranormal profits Profits earned by a natural monopolist not threatened by new entrants.

Introduction to market analysis

The role of markets and competition in health care has been brought to prominence in the discussion of health sector reforms all around the world. In many countries there is sizeable private activity in the health care sector. Under such circumstances, a market for health care is effectively operating and understanding the theory of markets may help governments to develop regulatory or incentive-based policies to ensure the appropriate operation of these markets. When a substantial private market exists in parallel with the public sector, it is important that public policies take account of the dynamics of the private market and the linkages between the public and private sectors.

A simple definition of a market is that it is a set of arrangements by which buyers and sellers are in contact to exchange goods and services. The market links demand (analysed in Chapters 3 and 4) and supply curves (Chapters 5 and 6).

In previous chapters you focused on the firm's production and costs. However, while you reviewed production bundles which were technically and economically efficient, you did not actually decide just how much the firm would eventually decide to produce. The cost curves you have reviewed can be used to develop a theory of the supply curve for a firm, but to understand how much is actually produced you also need to know something about the demand for the firm's product.

The level of output which a firm selects and the price which it charges for its product will depend on the structure of the market. Market structure can be thought of as a description of the behaviour of buyers and sellers, which will be determined largely by their size and number. One principle that distinguishes the various market structures is the degree of control that individual firms have over the price they are paid. Two cases that define the extreme forms of market structure are perfect competition and *monopoly*.

Although pure forms of these structures are uncommon, they are useful in showing the range of possible outcomes. Potential behaviour under some intermediate forms of market structure such as oligopoly will also be examined.

Perfect competition

The model of perfect competition is one where consumers are sovereign and firms are price takers; it is rarely seen in the world in its idealized form.

 Activity 7.1

From your existing knowledge, suggest and briefly describe four key conditions for perfect competition.

 Feedback

1 Large number of buyers and sellers, so that no actor alone can influence the price.

2 The good is *homogeneous* – all producers produce the same good, so that the market cannot be segmented on the basis of differences in goods.

3 There is perfect information – all buyers and sellers have information on all relevant variables such as prices and quality.

4 There are no barriers to entry or exit – a producer starts producing, buying necessary machinery, patents, or anything else, on the same terms as others already in the industry, and if they leave the market their assets can be readily sold or used for another purpose.

Although the market demand curve is usually downward-sloping, under perfect competition the demand curve facing an individual firm is horizontal. If the demand curve is horizontal, price (*p*) will be equal to *marginal revenue* (*MR*). Marginal revenue represents the change in the firm's total revenue resulting from a sale of one more unit of its product (see Figure 7.1).

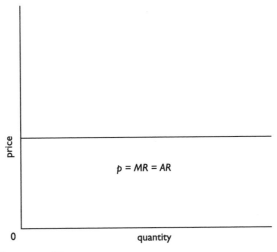

Figure 7.1 Perfect competition

Each extra good sold in a perfectly competitive market is sold at the market price. A horizontal demand curve implies that if the firm were to attempt to charge a price higher than the normal price, then it would not sell the product.

So far you have reviewed demand in a perfectly competitive market. What does the supply curve look like for an individual in a perfectly competitive market? If you consider the firm's marginal and average costs, the firm will be in *equilibrium* when marginal cost (*MC*) equals marginal revenue. This is because:

- the firm is a profit maximizer
- to the left of the point where $MR = MC$, $MR > MC$; thus any expansion in output will bring more revenue than it costs
- to the right of the point where $MR = MC$, $MR < MC$; thus by reducing the level of output, profits can be increased.

By shifting the price line it is possible to see how much the firm would supply at different prices and thus define the individual firm's supply curve. This coincides with the *MC* curve above the *AC* curve. The supply curve for the industry as a whole is simply the sum of individual supply curves (Figure 7.2).

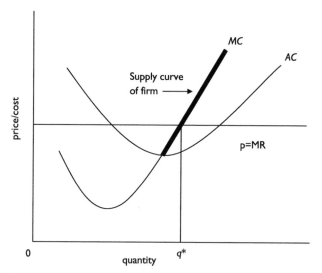

Figure 7.2 Supply curve of firm under perfect competition

If the price is greater than average cost, the firm will make a profit. By *normal profit* economists mean that economic profits are zero and the accounting profits just cover the opportunity cost of the owner's money and time. The cost curve incorporates the return that owners can normally get on their assets, and thus if owners are covering their costs, they are making normal profits. A 'normal' rate of return is included in costs, so profit implies an 'extra' rate of return above normal.

Profit is shown in the shaded area in Figure 7.3. If firms are making a profit, then there is an incentive for other firms to enter the industry, driving up supply and causing the price to fall. A new entrant will reduce profits in the industry to the level where they are zero. If profits become negative (Figure 7.4), then firms will leave the industry.

Thus in a perfectly competitive industry, in the long run, all firms will make a zero or normal profit – that is, they will make just sufficient profit to make it worth their while to stay in the industry.

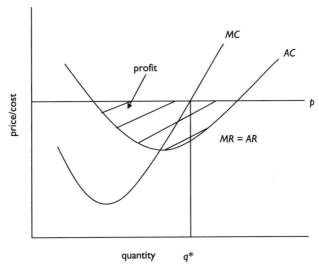

Figure 7.3 Profit scenario

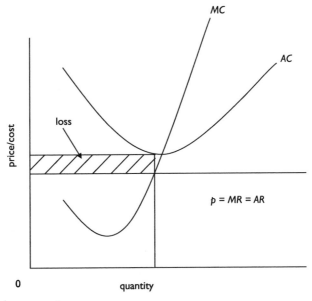

Figure 7.4 Loss scenario

Perfect competition and Pareto optimality

If you move from a partial equilibrium analysis (i.e. looking at one market in the economy) to a general equilibrium analysis, it can be shown that if all sectors of an economy are perfectly competitive and coordination is costless, then the resulting equilibrium in this idealized world will be Pareto-efficient. This is known as the *first fundamental theorem of welfare economics*.

In such a perfectly competitive economy, a number of marginal conditions are shown to hold, including:

*   *consumption* – consumers will consume at the point where their marginal rate of substitution between two goods is equal to the price ratio between those goods
*   *production* – firms will produce at the point where the marginal rate of technical substitution between the two factors is equal to the price ratio of those factors
*   the production sector plans are brought into line with the plans of consumers through the price signals of the market – thus *the market is coordinated as if by an 'invisible hand'*.

Activity 7.2

1   When will the firm be at equilibrium in the perfectly competitive market and why?
2   In a perfectly competitive market, at what point in the market will consumers fix their consumption and at what point will firms supply to the market?
3   Why do you think the price signals of the market would guide production with an 'invisible hand'?

Feedback

1 In the long run the firm will be at equilibrium in the perfectly competitive market when it is making zero profit, that is, when the marginal cost is equal to the price per unit. Costs just cover the opportunity costs of the entrepreneur's effort and time.

2 Consumers will choose to consume at that point where their marginal rate of substitution between two goods is equal to the price ratio between those goods, that is, $MRS_a/MRS_b = p_a/p_b$.

3 Although all consumers and producers may be free to act as they wish, the market conditions (i.e. the conditions of perfect competition) result in the plans of producers being brought into line with those of consumers. The metaphor of the 'invisible hand' goes back to the Scottish economist Adam Smith (1723–90) who in *An Inquiry into the Nature and Causes of the Wealth of Nations* (1776) laid the foundations of classical economic theory (see Smith 1970). He observed that though consumers and producers act in self-interest when making economic choices, the market forces lead the economy 'as if guided by an invisible hand' to mutually beneficial outcomes. Advocates of 'free markets' and *laissez-faire* economics often invoke Adam Smith and the notion of the 'invisible hand' in support.

There are a number of reasons why such arguments may be problematical in the case in health care markets. For instance, the conditions necessary for perfect competition are unlikely to prevail and, in addition, there may be public goods and externalities. It may also be the case that firms choose not to maximize profit. (For now you will proceed with an examination of different market forms without going into issues of market failure. These will be considered in Chapter 11.)

Even if the necessary conditions were to prevail, then the desirability of Pareto optimality as an end can be questioned, for reasons given in Chapter 1.

 Activity 7.3

1 Can you think of any markets that resemble perfect competition? What are their products or services? What characteristics do they have that make them resemble a perfect competition model?
2 Can you think of any health care markets that are perfectly competitive? What factors do you think might limit the ability of health care markets to have perfectly competitive characteristics?

 Feedback

1 Do the markets that you thought of meet all four of the assumptions of perfect competition? Are all firms price takers? Is there no product differentiation? Is information freely available to all market participants? Can firms freely enter or leave the market? Agriculture is sometimes put forward as an example of a highly competitive market, particularly in raw produce, since the scope for product differentiation is low. Although in theory these are important conditions for competition, in practice, competition in international agricultural markets is often undermined by political interests within high-income countries. In some manufacturing and service industries the conditions for perfect competition may also hold – particularly in low-technology industries (e.g. textile manufacture and unskilled service jobs).

2 It is difficult to think of health care markets that meet all four conditions for perfect competition:

- In some specialist areas there are very few suppliers, which means that prices rise well above marginal costs.
- The 'product' sold may vary in quality between suppliers.
- Health care consumers are not always fully informed.
- Barriers to entry exist in the form of qualifications needed by health care professionals.

Monopoly

In contrast to perfect competition, a monopolist is the sole supplier of the industry's product. A monopoly may be created by government action (e.g. the mail service), or it may be a natural one (e.g. a natural resource of limited supply) arising due to economies of scale.

As the monopolist is the sole supplier, the demand curve facing the industry is identical to the demand curve facing the individual firm, the monopolist. The demand curve is downward-sloping and therefore the marginal revenue curve is also downward-sloping (see Figure 7.5).

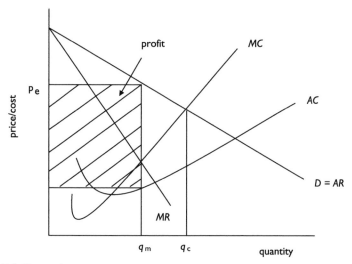

Figure 7.5 Monopoly

In order to maximize profits, the monopolist will also produce at the point (q_m) where $MR = MC$. The monopolist, unlike the producer in a perfectly competitive environment, is in the fortunate position of being able to set not only its own output levels but also its own price. The monopolist, having set a level of output, will set the price so as to maximize profit. As shown in Figure 7.5, the monopolist is likely to make a profit and, as there are no new entrants, will continue to make a profit even in the long run. However, it is not a foregone conclusion that profits will be made; this depends on the shape of both cost and demand curves.

In Figure 7.5, the monopoly price is presented by p_e, and profit is shown in the shaded area. This price is higher than the perfectly competitive price and the quantity is lower than the perfectly competitive quantity (q_c). In this situation, there is no supply curve, since there is only one price at which the monopolist is willing to supply output in this market. Thus you can see that a monopolist makes positive (*supranormal*) profits and it has been assumed that no entry takes place.

A potential strategy for the monopolist is to segment markets through price discrimination. As there are no competitors, monopolists are able to charge a higher price for the product to those with a greater willingness to pay. An example is the variety of prices that are used by train and airline companies for travel tickets. Price discrimination operates on the time of travel, class of travel, flexibility of travel and so on. The monopoly can claim higher prices from those consumers who are willing to pay more. This allows them to therefore cream off extra profits.

Activity 7.4

1   Are there any monopoly characteristics associated with health care?
2   Do single-price monopolies set output above or below what a perfectly competitive market would set?
3   Why are monopolies inefficient?

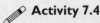 **Feedback**

1   In some cases there are close substitutes to health care, but in most cases there are probably not. For example, if someone has a cold or influenza then they could take symptom-controlling drugs. They could alternatively just spend some time in bed until the symptoms stop. In this case rest is a substitute for medication. However, with a disease like appendicitis there is no real substitute for surgical treatment.

Doctors, dentists and other health care professionals require a licence to practice. This licence is an example of a barrier to entry in the health care market. Patents are also barriers to entry because they prevent other manufacturers from producing a particular good. Patents are very common in the pharmaceutical industry. Consequently, it has been argued that allowing some degree of monopoly power encourages innovation within an industry. There may be examples of legal monopolies in health care in some countries as well.

Health care providers are not usually considered to be natural monopolies. Economies of scale exist only for small hospitals. It is unlikely, therefore, that a single provider can operate at a lower cost than would be achievable by several competing providers. However, in rural areas travel to other providers may be prohibitively expensive or not feasible for emergency conditions such that the local hospital is in effect a monopoly supplier for the local population.

2   A single price monopoly maximizes its profits at an output that is lower than the perfectly competitive industry output and a price that is higher. This is shown in Figure 7.5, where p_e is the equilibrium price, q_m is the quantity supplied in a monopoly market and q_c is the quantity that would otherwise be supplied in a competitive market.

3   Monopolies transform consumer surplus into producer surplus. However, the loss in consumer surplus is less than the gain in producer surplus. Therefore there is an overall loss to society (a deadweight loss).

It is sometimes suggested that monopolies are less able to achieve technical and economic efficiency. It is argued that their incentive to reduce cost is diminished because monopolies have very large profits already. On the other hand, the vast majority of research and development comes from very large suppliers, implying that these firms pay considerable attention to cost reduction. It has also been argued that the acquisition of monopoly power and thus supernormal profits can be a powerful incentive for firms to invest in research and development.

Contestability

It is often assumed that the number of competitors operating in a market is an indicator of the level of competition. The higher the number in a defined area, the higher the assumed level of competition. Indeed anti-trust (anti-monopoly) regulators in the USA have historically used various measures of industry concentration to make such judgements. However, it has been suggested that some industries may exhibit characteristics of competition even when there are a small number of firms (or indeed only one) operating in a market (Baumol 1982). This argument rests on the notion that such markets have reasonably low entry barriers and thus are influenced simply by the threat of potential entry of other firms. Therefore incumbents are constrained in the extent to which they are able to extract higher than normal profits through higher prices.

How applicable is the notion of contestability in health care? One feature of many forms of health care market is that there is often the requirement of some level of upfront investment. Such investment, sometimes referred to as *sunk cost*, may take the form of training (e.g. gaining qualifications) or equipment. The requirement for such investment can act as a barrier to entry (and exit) from such markets and can therefore be seen as an impediment to the attainment of contestability.

Depending on their regulatory and institutional context some health care markets, however, may have strong elements of contestability. For instance, in some low-income countries the retail pharmacy market can often be entered (as a supplier) with minimal investment. In many of these countries, drugs are sold over the counter in general stores or by unlicensed pharmacists.

 Activity 7.5

1 What sorts of health service costs could be considered 'sunk costs'?
2 What parts of the health care market might be more or less contestable?

 Feedback

1 Training might be considered a sunk cost, though to a certain extent training can be transferred across different specialties. Investments in specialized equipment and facilities, for example hospital equipment, might be hard to transfer to another industry and therefore constitute barriers to entry into the health sector.

2 Markets for primary care could be considered contestable, to the extent that doctors from other fields could potentially enter (though professional restrictions requiring specialized training could erode this contestability), and the premises and equipment required are not highly specialized and could be used for other purposes. Pharmaceutical retailing could be a contestable market if leases for shop premises can easily be terminated and transferred to other retail activities, and unsold stock sold to other providers (e.g. hospitals).

Health care markets

Because of the lack of feasibility of patients travelling long distances when in need of urgent attention and the non-tradeable nature of health care, certain providers with large economies of scale may be in a monopoly position. How should government attempt to intervene (if at all) to offset this? Where there are cases of natural monopoly (e.g. electricity generation, gas distribution), government may seek to regulate by controlling levels of profitability or prices. In health care, however, the drawbacks to these approaches are fairly self-evident; there is little point in government controlling prices or profits unless it can also control quality or costs. The great heterogeneity of health care services and the difficulties involved in measuring quality mean that such approaches are uncommon.

 Activity 7.6

Now that you have learned about the characteristics of perfectly competitive, monopolistic and contestable markets, think of markets in the health sector in your country.

What characteristics of each of the types of market models considered do they have? Remember that markets are the exchange of goods and services. These could include treatments, health care workforce, and catering services, for example.

 Feedback

Although you will find a large range of different types of health care markets, few will be perfectly competitive. An example you might think of is generic painkillers sold over the counter (i.e. not on prescription), such as paracetamol, which are produced in large quantities by many different firms. Consumers may make their choice based on price. Most health care markets tend to be monopolistic or oligopolistic. You may look at market segmentation in terms of provider qualification, geographical area, level of care, fee levels charged and so on. For example, specialist care centres need specific human resources and are tailored to the needs of relatively small patient numbers, creating barriers to entry for new providers. Other examples of monopolies are health facilities that are the only providers in remote areas. Competition between providers is usually greater in urban areas where multiple providers are attracted by the demand from the middle classes. You may also consider who dominates different sectors of health care markets – modern or traditional practitioners, allopathic or homeopathic medicines, private or public providers. You will also have found that health care markets are contestable: a drug firm may lower prices even before the patent protection of its product expires as it fears competition from other drug companies which are preparing to enter the market. Health labour markets can also be contestable, for instance allowing other professionals to provide comparable services: think of the potential competition for orthopaedic surgeons and physiotherapists when, for example, osteopaths and chiropractors are considered as potential competitors.

Monopsony

A similar market analysis takes place in the situation where you have one buyer rather than one seller. Figure 7.6 illustrates this situation. In this context, the supply curve shows the amount of output different suppliers are willing to provide at different prices to the one buyer. In a competitive market, demand would be equated to supply. However, if there is only one buyer, the monopsonist will produce until $MR = MC$. In this case, the buyer's MC is different from the industry supply curve. This is because although in the industry the supplier is willing to sell output at different prices, there is only one buyer who pays the same price for all the outputs purchased (e.g. even though the supplier is willing to provide additional output at a higher price, the buyer has to buy even the first unit of output at this higher price). Thus the buyer equates MC to MR and the resulting equilibrium is one where the output sold is less than in a perfectly competitive outcome and the price paid is also less.

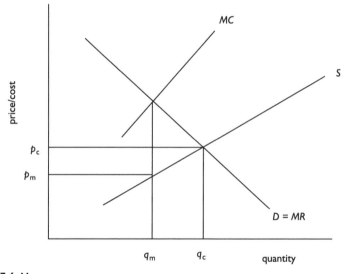

Figure 7.6 Monopsony

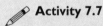

Activity 7.7

Can you think of any examples of monopsony in the health sector?

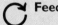

Feedback

Several hospitals may combine their buying power to achieve better contracts with suppliers. Several insurance companies may negotiate joint contracts with providers to obtain discounts. Monopsony is even more pronounced if there is only one single purchaser of services, as in publicly funded health systems.

So far in this chapter you have learned about monopolies, monopsonies and contestable markets. You have examined their relevance to the health care sector. You will now look at examples of imperfect competition.

Imperfect competition

Between the two extremes of perfect competition and pure monopoly there is a range of market forms.

Oligopoly and game theory

The key feature of an *oligopoly* is that the decision made by one firm depends on the decision made by other firms, that is, there is a high degree of inter-dependence between firms. Firms therefore can only decide upon their own best strategy in the light of what they know about other firms. Many different possible models exist, based principally on different assumptions about other firms in the market.

Game theory attempts to model the behaviour of firms by seeing them as players in a game. The classic game is that of the Prisoner's dilemma. This game is usually illustrated by an example in which two prisoners (A and B) are each offered separately the opportunity to confess to a crime. They are, however, locked in separate rooms and therefore have no means of communicating with one another. If both confess, they are given a sentence of 3 years each (punishment for mutual non-cooperation (defection), P). If, however, prisoner A confesses but prisoner B does not, then B receives 7 years (sucker's payoff, S) and A receives no sentence for turning informant (temptation payoff, T). On the other hand, if the prisoners manage to cooperate with one another and both do not confess, then they each receive a sentence of 1 year (reward payoff, R). Table 7.1 shows the payoff matrix for this problem.

Table 7.1 Prisoners' dilemma game

		Prisoner A	
		Confess	Not confess
Prisoner B	Confess	3,3	7,0
	Not confess	0,7	1,1

There are two formal conditions for a prisoners' dilemma game (Axelrod 1988). First, each prisoner faces a set of payoffs ordered in the following manner (from worst to best in terms of years in jail) $S>P>R>T$.

The second condition is that $T+S>R+R$ so that the option of each player in taking turns at exploiting the other in successive games yields a lower payoff in total (or in this case, a greater number of years in jail) than mutual cooperation. In any case, this is unlikely to occur if, as set out in the conditions, prisoners are unable to communicate.

In these games, regardless of the choice made by the other player, non-cooperation (defection) represents the dominant strategy for each player. This means that each player is always better off confessing regardless of what the other player does. A Nash equilibrium occurs when each player pursues this (presented in bold in Table 7.1) and represents the situation where each player can do no better for themselves in choosing an alternative option. Such a strategy, which involves each player pursuing their individually optimal strategy, however, is not optimal collectively since each could do better if they cooperated with one another (1 year rather than 3 years).

Some of the early applications of game theory involving these types of models were in political science, looking, for instance, at issues of diplomacy and the nuclear arms race. Their value is that they analyse the outcomes of decisions made interactively between a number of parties. As a consequence, games have also been fruitfully applied to the analysis of firms' decisions about outputs in the market. The number of times these decisions are to be made and firms' beliefs about each other become critical factors determining outcomes. A substantial part of the literature looks at collusion, where there is an explicit attempt by the different firms in the industry to coordinate their pricing and output strategies so that together they can reap monopolistic profits. In urban markets dominated by a small number of hospitals, for example, it is conceivable that they might try to fix prices. However, as shown by the experience of cartels such as OPEC during the 1980s, formal collusion through cartels is very vulnerable to price cutting among members.

Another way in which these types of markets can be configured involves collusion whereby one dominant firm acts as a leader in terms of pricing decisions.

Asymmetric information

The presence of asymmetric information between producer and consumer may also give rise to forms of imperfect competition. For example, consider a situation where products are not homogeneous and consumers have preferences for different products. However, there are likely to be search costs associated with finding their preferred product. Consumers will only invest in search activity up to the point where the expected marginal benefit of a search is equal to the marginal cost. Under such conditions, consumers may not search the whole market and hence producers may retain a degree of market power. The smaller the search cost, the better informed the consumer will be and the more closely the model will approximate perfect competition.

Summary

You have learned about the theories relating to different market structures, from the extremes of perfect competition and monopoly to a range of alternative models. You have looked at how different market structures will have implications for the demand and supply of a product, and the significance of these market structures in particular for the operation of health care markets.

References

Axelrod R (1988) The problem of co-operation, in Cowen T (ed) *The Theory of Market Failure. A Critical Examination* pp. 237–54. Fairfax, VA: George Mason University Press:

Baumol WJ (1982) Contestable markets: an uprising in the theory of industry structure. *American Economic Review* 72: 1–15.

Smith A (1970) *An Inquiry into the Nature and Causes of the Wealth of Nations.* Harmondsworth: Penguin.

8 | Behaviour of health care providers

Overview

In the previous chapter you learned about different types of market structure and their implications in terms of prices, outputs, profits and efficiency. You explored the idealized model of perfect competition as an extreme in the range of possibilities. The underlying assumptions which generated a perfectly competitive market structure were discussed, and it was emphasized that one of the implicit assumptions was the notion that the firm is a profit-maximizing entity. The standard model suggested that competition (or the threat of competition – contestability) was beneficial for consumers in that it led to lower prices and greater supply.

However, you also saw that there might be good reasons why competition in markets for health care does not take the same form as competition in other sectors of the economy. One important issue is that health care providers may not adhere to the simple model of the profit-maximizing firm that is used in conventional economic theory. This chapter introduces you to some of the alternative models that have been developed to understand health care provider behaviour.

Learning objectives

After working through this session, you should be able to:

- discuss the extent to which health care providers may be motivated by factors other than profit maximization
- describe three models of provider motivation and their predictions about provider behaviour
- assess the assumptions about provider behaviour which underlie hospital reforms, and what the reforms imply for the appropriate ways to model hospital behaviour.

Key terms

Managerial utility function A function that states that managerial utility is determined by salary, security, power and status.

Procedural rationality Where agents do not necessarily succeed in maximizing their own goals but give each decision deliberation that is appropriate to its relative importance.

> **Revenue maximization** Maximizing the amount the firm earns by selling goods or services in a given period of time – this is different from profits, which are the excess of revenues over costs.
>
> **Substantive rationality** Where rational agents maximize the achievement of their own goals, given existing constraints.

Introduction

A common assumption underlying the basic analyses of market structures is that of the firm as a profit maximizer. Such an assumption can be seen to be the opposite side of the coin to that of utility maximization among consumers – as discussed in Chapter 1. The notion of rationality as encapsulated in such models of maximizing behaviour is important in making tractable conventional (or neoclassical) forms of analysis. However, the value of economic models should be based not on their analytical elegance but on how well they describe and predict reality. This therefore begs the question: are models of maximizing behaviour realistic? If not, are there alternative models of behaviour? This chapter focuses specifically on alternative models of provider behaviour in health care and reviews alternatives. (In relation to the consumer side and the assumption of utility maximization, the next chapter dealing with the issues of consumerism touch upon alternative motivations.)

Perhaps the best-recognized instance where the motive of profit maximization is seen not to apply is when the managers of organizations have alternative motives to those of the owners (in the context of private companies) or of the organization in general (particularly in the public sector where certain social objectives may be seen as the guiding objectives of the organization). In these cases the problems resemble those that can beset the doctor–patient relationship, namely, imperfect agency (as discussed in Chapter 4). In relation to the private sector, particularly in corporations where management is separated from ownership, McPake *et al.* (2002) identify salary, security, power and status as variables that may influence the behaviour of managers. In such instances, it is possible that managers may be more attracted to revenue than to profit maximization as an objective. They also cite some previous research in the USA that identifies objectives of hospital managers such as level of emergency stand-by capacity, total admissions, case mix and practice style (Hornbrook and Goldfarb 1983).

In relation to public sector managers, Jan (2000) employs the assumption of *budget* maximization but also highlights a number of other possibilities: discretionary budget maximization (which is total budget minus the production cost of undertaking core activities); lifetime rewards as opposed to the prevailing level of reward; and 'the quiet life' (i.e. some managers may seek to minimize effort). In some cases, there may be value to a manager in gaining a reputation as a 'hatchetman'. This would then imply the opposite motivation to budget maximization.

Activity 8.1

Think of an organization where ownership and management are separated – for example, where the owner of a firm has employed a manager.

1 Suggest some examples of the key motivating factors that influence the managers at work.
2 What organizational objectives other than maximizing profit might the manager have?
3 How does the separation of ownership and management translate into the public sector context? Can you think of circumstances where public sector managers might be motivated by profit maximization?

Feedback

1 There are many intrinsic and extrinsic factors motivating people at work, such as payment, professional success, career prospect, status, power and self-actualization.

2 Organizational objectives other than profit maximization may include revenue maximization, achieving performance targets, or, in the case of health care organizations, meeting the health care needs of a defined population or meeting treatment targets agreed in contracts. While profit maximization is a driving force in private sector health care and the drugs and supply industry, it is not usually a goal in public sector organizations.

3 We can think of the owners in the public sector as being the government, with the managers operating the health care facilities. While the government is usually not trying to pursue profits from its health care facilities, in some circumstances provider managers might act as profit maximizers, for instance if they receive user fee revenue which the facility is able to retain and use to pay staff bonuses or improve working conditions.

Behavioural theory

These variations from the conventional assumption of firms being profit maximizers have their roots in the work of Herbert Simon (1959) and can be broadly categorized as behavioural theories. Simon argued that the conventional way of examining firms was to assume that their behaviour was guided by notions of substantive rationality, that is, was based on the behaviour of agents who would seek to achieve the maximization of a certain identified objective subject to given constraints. He argued, however, that in practice individual agents' capacity to act in this manner was bounded by factors such as informational constraints and therefore they tended to be guided more by rule-of-thumb measures (procedural rationality).

By analytically separating the behaviour and motivations of the individual and the firm, this type of framework introduces the possibility of there being an inconsistency between the interests of individual decision makers and the objectives of the firm as well as inconsistency among the interests of decision makers within the firm. This framework thus introduces into the analysis factors such as the relative power of actors and the institutional context of decision making – issues that tend to be overlooked in the conventional production function approaches (see Chapter 5).

Activity 8.2

Identify one or more reforms to hospitals in your country. These might include: changes to the way hospitals are paid (fee-for-service (FFS), global budgets, prospective payment mechanisms such as diagnosis-related groups); measures to increase the autonomy of hospitals by allowing them greater freedom to set policies and prices; financing reform which allows hospitals to introduce charges for services and retain these for use in the hospital; quality improvement systems such as hospital accreditation.

What do these reforms assume about hospital objectives? What sort of model of hospital behaviour underlies the reforms?

How do these reforms alter the incentives facing hospitals? Are they likely to change the balance of power between doctors and managers?

What are anticipated outcomes of the reforms? Is there a risk of any unanticipated negative effects?

Feedback

The key here is to think about whether there are unrealistic assumptions regarding the motivations of key actors implicit in these reforms. Is it assumed, for instance, that the policies to contract out services to the private sector will be implemented in such a way that the individuals responsible for the tendering process ensure that the best contracts (from the point of view of the organization) are awarded, and are there incentives in place for these contracts to be properly monitored? Of course, this task is also complicated in many situations where policy reforms create winners and losers – the implementation of an initiative might mean shifting resources away from an existing programme. In these cases the question arises whether it is possible to achieve reform in the face of potential opposition from those who would lose out, such as the managers of the programmes that lose funding. (Chapter 12 examines similar issues in relation to regulation.)

Three models of hospital behaviour

Three models were developed in the 1970s primarily in the USA particularly in relation to private non-profit types of hospital. In generalizing some of the lessons gained from these models, it is necessary to take into account the different objectives and constraints faced by decision makers within hospital organizations in other contexts (e.g. public hospitals in public systems).

Pauly and Redisch (1973) assume that hospital resources are controlled by doctors. The main predictions of their model relate to the optimal staffing level and the effects on prices and output of services. The predictions of the model depend on whether the outcome is cooperative or non-cooperative (which itself depends on the number of doctors). In the cooperative case, the model predicts that doctors will act as a cartel, controlling their own numbers, keeping prices high and output lower. In the non-cooperative case, the model predicts that the cartel may break down because of free-riding by some doctors.

Newhouse (1970) assumes that hospitals are controlled by their managers, whose utility function includes both quantity and quality of output. This model predicts that hospitals are willing to sacrifice quantity for quality, leading to a bias towards high quality services, duplication of equipment, and choice of capital-intensive medical procedures.

Harris (1977) addresses both managers' and doctors' utility – proposing that the hospital can be understood as made up of two separate firms which are interacting to produce health care. However, like Newhouse's managers, the doctors are motivated by both quantity and quality. Harris's model predicts that this leads to excess capacity and a tendency to expand facilities (subject to the budget constraint).

 Activity 8.3

Think about how the ideas in these models apply to the hospital sector in your country. In particular, how might the method of remuneration for doctors affect behaviour? What other issues might come into play?

 Feedback

The key is in distinguishing the differences in incentives between methods of remuneration that give doctors some stake in the performance of the organization (profit sharing, fee-for-service (FFS)) and those that do not (most notably, fixed wages). However, there are numerous other issues that will affect behaviour, such as whether doctors have admitting privileges; whether hospitals are owned by doctors; whether doctors are allowed to admit private patients into public hospitals; whether private hospitals are for profit or non-profit (and how this affects their objectives); and how hospitals receive their funds (e.g. from government, from insurers, from out-of-pocket payments).

In addition, in low- and middle-income countries the nature and effectiveness of monitoring and regulatory systems within hospitals may be relevant. In such settings it is often the case that the capacity of organizations, particularly within the public sector, to undertake such activities is limited by major resource constraints.

McPake *et al.* (2002) examine some of the implications of this for health policy:

"Why do we want to better understand the motivations and therefore behaviour of hospitals or other health service providers? Much of the content of health policy is designed to influence the behaviour of health service providers. For example, changes in hospital reimbursement mechanisms have usually been designed in order to change the incentives facing hospitals and therefore their behaviour – perhaps on the assumption that provider institutions are profit or revenue maximizing. The introduction of separation between purchasers and providers seems to assume that providers will respond to market forces by trying to improve the quality and efficiency with which they offer services – but why should they, if profit maximization is not their objective? Even interventions such as in-service training programmes designed to improve the appropriateness of care provided, or attempts to improve management information systems, assume a particular set of motivations. In these cases, perhaps the assumption is that hospital decision makers will strive to make the most technically appropriate decisions if only they are provided with the necessary technical skills and information – in other words, that they are the perfect agents of their patients, or even of society . . . all these assumptions seem rather simplistic . . . In order to manage incentives, it is important to understand motivation."

 Activity 8.4

Think back over the models of non-profit-maximizing hospital behaviour discussed in this chapter and make brief notes on the strengths and weaknesses of applying the theory of the firm to the hospital sector.

 Feedback

All models have their limitations as they can only predict certain aspects of the economic behaviour in the hospital sector. Some of the models take insufficient account of the internal structure by putting too much emphasis on the role of the manager or of the doctors. A key problem of transferring the theory of the firm to the hospital is that prices play only a limited role in allocative decisions and that behaviour is dominated by non-market relations between the actors. Other problems which make it difficult to establish a general economic model of the hospital are related to measuring performance and taking account of the complexity of organizational structure.

Summary

You have learned about managerial and behavioural theories of the firm, including substantive and procedural rationality. In addition, you have learned about explicit non-profit-maximizing behaviour in the hospital and you have considered three models used to describe hospital behaviour: the hospital as a doctors' cooperative, the quantity/quality non-profit theory and the Harris model.

References

Harris JE (1977) The internal organization of hospitals: some economic implications. *Bell Journal of Economics* 8: 467–82.
Hornbrook MC and Goldfarb MG (1983) A partial test of a hospital behavioral model. *Social Science & Medicine* 17: 667–80.
Jan S (2000) Institutional considerations in priority setting: transactions cost perspective on PBMA. *Health Economics* 9: 631–41.

McPake B, Kumaranayake L and Normand C (2002) *Health Economics: An International Perspective*. London: Routledge.

Newhouse JP (1970) Toward a theory of non-profit institutions: an economic model of the hospital. *American Economic Review* 60: 64–74.

Pauly M and Redisch M (1973) The not-for-profit hospital as a physician's cooperative. *American Economic Review* 63: 87–100.

Simon HA (1959) Theories of decision-making in economics and behavioral science. *American Economic Review* 49: 797–825.

9 What is the evidence of competition on the consumer and provider sides?

Overview

You have so far looked at different models of how a hospital or firm may behave in terms of making decisions. You will now examine the behaviour of the consumer of health services. The aim of this chapter is to consider the evidence relating to whether patients in health care markets act like consumers in other markets, particularly whether patients are willing and able to make health care choices on the basis of sensitivity to cost and quality of services. In the second part of this chapter you will turn to market structure and examine the theory and evidence linking market structure with market performance measures, such as price and cost.

Learning objectives

After working through this chapter you should be able to:

- discuss the extent to which patients in the health care market act like consumers in other markets and how this might in turn affect provider behaviour
- describe current evidence of consumer behaviour in the health care market
- outline the use of the Hirshfeld–Herfindahl Index and describe ways of measuring competition between health care providers
- critically assess the theory underlying market competition and how this is studied empirically.

Key terms

Consumerism The readiness of consumers of health care services (patients) to exercise their choices in markets, actively seeking out and comparing information on price and quality.

Hirschman-Herfindahl Index A measure of the degree of market concentration, aimed at estimating the competitiveness of the market, and defined as the sum of squared market shares of all firms in the industry.

n-firm concentration ratio A measure of the degree of market concentration, aimed at estimating the competitiveness of the market, and defined as the aggregate market share of the n largest firms in the industry.

Introduction

Models of provider competition are based upon different assumptions about the health care consumer. For example, you may assume that consumers are not sensitive to price but judge a service by easily discernible aspects of quality (such as equipment available). A different assumption may be that price matters more than quality in choosing a provider – for example, that patients are price-conscious when buying a medicine. You may also make certain assumptions as to the behaviour of patients during a consultation with a practitioner. There is a continuum between seeing a patient as a passive subject who is unwilling to question a provider's authority and an active and well-informed consumer of health care who makes choices between different providers, for example, by getting a second opinion.

Consumer behaviour in the health care market

How consumers behave in the health care market is an empirical question. In different cultures, individuals may approach health care very differently. Although many of the recent market-oriented reforms explicitly avoid placing the consumer in the role of the primary purchaser of health care, consumers nonetheless play a role in promoting competition. In low-income countries, where there are rarely institutional purchasers to act on behalf of consumers, the role of consumer behaviour is critical.

A number of studies in the UK (Higgins and Wiles 1992), the USA (Hibbard and Weeks 1987) and Australia (Donaldson et al. 1991; Lupton 1997) have explored consumer behaviour. On the whole, results suggest that patients are disinclined to act as 'consumers'. For example, with respect to knowledge, Higgins and Wiles found that the major reason given by patients in the private sector for seeking care privately rather than publicly was the length of waiting lists in the public sector, but when questioned closely, few knew how long the expected waiting time was. Of these private patients, 62% did not know how much the treatment would cost and 70% of those insured did not know whether any co-payment would be necessary. In another study, the major reason found for selecting a general practitioner (GP) in the UK was proximity; respondents often said that their GP was the closest to their home. However, the researchers often found another practice even closer to their residence.

Hibbard and Weeks (1987) considered three aspects of consumer behaviour:

- knowledge – both current knowledge and willingness to seek new information
- attitudes – particularly with respect to consumers' willingness to use their own independent judgements
- behaviour – especially individual sensitivity to cost and quality.

The level of 'consumerist' behaviour exhibited by patients is probably strongly influenced by the type of health care system to which they are accustomed. For instance, in predominantly private systems insurance companies may restrict the providers and the services from which a patient may choose.

Lupton et al. (1991) conducted a cross-sectional survey of patients seeking care from a GP in Australia. The following describes their findings.

Consumerism, reflectivity and the medical encounter

The key issues identified were those relating to the ability and the motivation of the respondents to actively evaluate their GPs, and their tendency towards blind loyalty towards their regular GPs. Although appearing to have chosen their doctor in a casual manner, only a small minority of respondents reported ever changing to another doctor or considering such a move. The majority of respondents adhered to a satellite rather than a pluralist model of health care use, preferring to return to their regular GP for care whenever possible, rather than choosing to seek attention from other GPs or alternate primary health care providers. Alternate providers were accessed only if the regular GP was unavailable. Respondents did not, for the most part, actively 'shop around' to try out or compare the services of alternate primary health care providers. Accessibility issues seemed unimportant to this sample when choosing a GP. Some respondents were aware that there is asymmetry of information between patient and doctor which acts as a barrier to effective evaluation of the doctor's service by the patient. It was pointed out that habit and trust seemed to prevent most people from being able to evaluate their GP's services. Similarly, although the majority of respondents thought that most people would have the ability to evaluate doctors' services, many answers justified this belief by citing elements of faith and trust rather than 'rational' judgement, emphasising the significance of 'gut feelings' and 'instinct'.

. . . The results of this exploratory survey indicate that assumptions that Australian patients are behaving consumeristically may be inappropriate. The majority of respondents did not approach their choice of GP as ideal type consumers but rather demonstrated a need to feel protected from the effects of the free market. These results lead to the conclusion that patients prefer to keep themselves in a state of 'blissful ignorance' rather than behaving in a consumerist manner. Many respondents mentioned the 'trust' and 'faith' they had in their regular doctor, and mentioned his or her 'dedication to the profession'. These sentiments evoke a common image of a GP similar to that characterising members of the clergy: someone who is bound by duty to help his or her clients, who is benevolent, who is caring and friendly but who remains in a position of authority at all times, in whom one can place all one's trust.

 Activity 9.1

To what extent do you think consumerism plays a role in your own health care system?

 Feedback

The extent to which consumerist behaviour is emerging in your country's health care system will rest on a range of political, social and cultural factors. For instance, a major consideration may be whether patients purchase services directly, through a third party such as an insurer (in which case there may be another issue as to whether there is a significant co-payment involved) or receive them free. It may be the case that consumerist behaviour is more likely the more directly the consumer is involved in purchasing care.

Lupton et al. (1991) found evidence in in-depth interviews with a subsample of the study population that the role people take depends on their personal circumstances. In the medical encounter, people may pursue the 'active consumer' and the 'passive patient' positions simultaneously or variously depending on the context.

Measuring market structure

Most theories of imperfect competition assume that market structure has an impact upon the way in which the market operates: market structure (the number of sellers in the market, their degree of product differentiation and the cost structure) determines conduct (which consists of price, research and development, investment, advertising and so on) and so yields market performance (efficiency, ratio of price to marginal cost, profits). This is commonly known as the structure–conduct–performance paradigm.

This paradigm has been very influential, and economists have developed measures of market concentration in order to operationalize and test the theory with empirical data. The simplest measure is the n-firm concentration ratio, which measures the aggregate market share of the n largest firms in the industry (n is usually 3 or 5). However, this measure only considers the n largest firms in the industry and is insensitive to the way these shares are distributed across the n firms.

Alternatively, there is the Hirschman–Herfindahl Index (HHI), which is defined as the sum of the squared market shares of all firms in the industry. The value of the HHI ranges from 0 (large number of competitors all with small market shares) to 1 (single monopoly supplier).

More recently there has been criticism of the structure–conduct–performance paradigm from the perspective that the firm's conduct can be targeted at changing the structure of the industry. For example, advertising strategies may explicitly aim to concentrate market power in the hands of fewer competitors. Nonetheless concentration measures such as these are still widely used both to study market behaviour and in legal cases where industries are challenged for behaving monopolistically.

The relationship between market structure and market power (ability to influence the terms on which transactions are made) can vary. As discussed in Chapter 7, it can be the degree of contestability as opposed to the number of providers that is crucial to understanding the power exerted by individual firms.

Another problem with looking at market structure is the whole issue of how to define a market. Market definitions need to address the boundaries of both the product and the geographical area.

The following passage from Nakamba *et al.* (2002) discusses markets for hospital services in Zambia.

Markets for hospital services in Zambia

As part of the autonomy arrangements for hospitals, they are allowed to generate additional revenue from the sale of private inpatient and outpatient services provided in designated 'high cost' wards. In theory these services are distinguished by higher quality hotel services. High cost services, therefore, can be considered a separate product, with services provided in private facilities acting as closer substitutes than those in lower level or other public facilities. A different market definition may therefore be applied to 'high cost' services. Despite all of the complexity in defining product markets, the analysis that follows relies on fairly crude product definitions due to the absence of disaggregated utilization data. Thus, we look primarily at inpatient services provided by officially recognized hospitals, and at the distinction between low cost and high cost services.

Defining the geographic boundary is the second key step in the patient flow approach. Three methods have been used: geopolitical boundaries, distances from hospitals and patient origin data ... Despite the obvious limitations, we have taken the administrative boundary of the province as the primary geographic dimension to our market definition. We have chosen to examine the hospital service markets in the Central, Lusaka and Copperbelt provinces, because these provinces have a relatively greater number of non-public facilities. They therefore represent an upper bound on the level of competition that can be expected in Zambia, and are thus important for understanding the operation of hospital markets ...

While accepting the empirical evidence that actual patient flow between provinces is limited, we have chosen to aggregate two provinces (Central and Lusaka) into a single market, 'Midlands'. The justification for this aggregation lies in the notion of potential competition and contestability. The distance between the two main cities in these provinces, Lusaka and Kabwe, is relatively small and easily travelled by car or public transport. It is therefore likely that patients in the Central province perceive the Lusaka hospitals to belong to their choice set. We have also been guided by local knowledge and the fact that the markets are perceived to operate as one.

 Activity 9.2

   1 Assess the method of Nakamba et al. for measuring the product and geographical markets for hospital services. What are the main problems with it? How would you modify or improve on it in your setting?

   2 How would a narrower definition of the product market (e.g. particular surgical procedures) affect the measure of market competition?

 Feedback

   1 Any analysis of health care markets should take a consumer perspective and analyse how economic behaviour of the key actors in a defined local market affects access to care. It should assess the patterns of patient flows, the degree of provider concentration and examine how the actors try to gain market dominance. A critical aspect of the analysis is to establish a clear definition of the market in terms of geographical boundaries and products as this may affect the conclusions drawn about the level of market concentration.

   2 Narrower product markets (e.g. ophthalmic surgery) will usually be more concentrated than broader markets (e.g. general surgery).

Market concentration

Despite the possible significance of contestability, a number of studies have looked at market concentration as evidence of competition, particularly in relation to the provision of hospital services. Understanding market concentration levels may be of importance to health service planners and managers as a signal of technical and allocative efficiency of hospital services and resource provision in an area. It may also act as an indicator of managerial, staff and consumer behaviour in an area. For example, why is hospital X finding it difficult to recruit staff? Which hospital do patients in region Z use and why?

Linking market structure and outcomes

The following extract by Carol Propper and Neil Soderlund (1998) examines competition in the British NHS internal market and its effect on costs and prices.

Market structure and prices

In 1991, the UK Government introduced into its National Health Service (NHS) a 'quasi-market' for hospital services. Newly established purchasers, District Health Authorities (DHAs) and General Practice Fund Holders (GPFHs) were allocated budgets and were required to purchase care from autonomous hospitals. At least one, if not the primary intention was to improve the efficiency of health care providers through competition . . .

Competition might manifest itself in a number of ways. In the short run, lower prices might be charged for similar products, or higher quality products might be offered for the same price. Both phenomena would in turn be expected to put pressure on quality-adjusted unit costs in proportion to the degree of competition for the services concerned. The impact of the reforms with regard to productivity should thus be evidenced by the degree to which competition affects observed prices and quality of services offered with fairly immediate effect, with a slightly delayed impact on costs. In the long run, we would expect competition to impact on market structure through changes in the size of institutions, degree of specialization, exit of unsuccessful players and entry of new ones . . .

The traditional view of competition is that its effect is to lower prices and costs for a given service. The existence of rivals means providers must reduce price to attract business, so competition limits the economic inefficiencies associated with monopoly power. This view underlies the rationale for the introduction of competition in health care markets in general, and the creation of the NHS internal market in particular. Given this argument, we would expect prices and costs to be lower in more competitive markets – those geographical areas in which there are more providers of health care.

This simple model of competition in the NHS has been challenged from a number of angles. Chalkey and Malcolmson (1995) . . . have suggested that competition may not be needed in the internal market to reduce allocative inefficiency where there is bilateral monopoly (a single provider and a single purchaser). They show that if the purchaser and provider have sufficient information about each other – in particular they know each other's reservation price for services of known quality – then bilateral monopoly will be efficient. In other words, competition is not needed to reduce inefficiencies. But the argument rests on the assumption that both parties are well informed. Furthermore, the situation they describe – that of bilateral monopoly between a single purchaser and a single provider – is not the norm in the internal market. While each local market is characterized by a limited number of purchasers and providers, there is usually more than one provider, and given the rise in the number of GPFHs during the years 1991–1997, there is certainly more than one purchaser. The precise relationship between the number of sellers (competition) and prices and efficiency will then be more difficult to determine.

Dawson (1994) . . . has also criticized the traditional view of purchaser–provider relationships which postulates a simple inverse relationship between the degree of competition in a geographic area and posted prices for services as being unrealistic. Given the limited number of both buyers and sellers in any geographic area, she argues that posted prices are largely irrelevant in negotiations. Instead contracts are determined by an opaque process of bargaining that is highly context-specific and has long term collaborative objectives. Neither party has any interest in disclosing real price information, and so any form of regulation based on posted prices, such as the 'cost equals price' rule currently in place in the NHS . . . is likely to be inappropriate.

Her argument applies particularly to DHA contracts with major providers, where large blocks of activity to be delivered in a specific geographic area are being negotiated, and both monopoly and monopsony power would be expected to be important bargaining tools. Her argument implies that posted prices offer little real guidance to negotiated prices, but this does not necessarily imply that competition has no impact on actual negotiated prices.

In reality, it is likely that both posted-price competition, and secret negotiation for block contracts operate simultaneously, but for different types of activity and buyers. So prices may be some guide to the impact of competition. In addition, the extent of monopoly power for providers, and hence their price levels, might also vary according to the nature of the service, the mix of purchasers concerned, types of contracting arrangement, and the amount of spare capacity amongst competitors. For example, while emergency services must be provided within a certain time, for other services patients may be prepared to trade-off travel time against other costs. Consequently, there may be more competition for elective services than for emergency services. Similarly, some purchasers, for example GPFHs, may be more willing to shop around for care . . . than DHAs, for whom consistency of supply of services in a given geographical area is of highest priority . . . On the other hand, once DHAs have secured consistent supply of the majority of services required, they might be prepared to shop around for specialized, out-of-district, extra contractual services, for which there are potentially a number of suppliers. Related to this, where purchasers are seeking to buy care for an individual patient, prices are posted in advance, and are easily compared, suggesting that price competition will be easier in the purchasing of care outside of bulk contracts. By the same token, where providers have assurance that their fixed costs will be met by bulk contracts, prices for residual activities need only cover marginal cost, and there is thus significant potential for discounting should competition force this. The larger the amount of spare capacity that competitors have, the greater we would expect the competition in this 'residual capacity' market to be . . .

In addition to a firm theoretical basis, we also require a number of market prerequisites for price competition to be identified in the NHS. First, there needs to be more than one provider of services in each geographic area. The NHS internal market was built on the foundation of a centrally planned hospital system, where extensive efforts went into avoiding duplication of services. We might thus expect there to be limited scope for competition among hospitals. But an examination of the distribution of hospitals in the UK indicates that relatively few providers do not have another provider located within a 30-minute travel distance . . .

Second, the operation of markets requires that providers have both the incentives to compete with other providers, and the managerial independence to respond to competition by lowering prices and cutting costs appropriately. On the provider side, the establishment of trust hospitals has given them some of these freedoms, although trusts are still not allowed to retain surpluses that they might make, so pure profit incentives might be somewhat attenuated . . . But the actions of hospitals remain heavily regulated by the Department of Health. At least one of the regulations is expressly intended to limit price competition, the regulation that hospitals price care at cost with no cross-subsidies . . . (the 'price equals cost' rule). But additional non-profit gains can still be made by successful managers; examples are performance-related pay rises, reputational benefits, and improved working conditions generated by diverting operational surpluses into their own departmental budgets . . .

The main results from the studies reviewed by Propper and Soderlund (1998) can be summarized as follows:

- High levels of price variability between providers that are not explained solely by variation in cost suggest that NHS pricing rules have not had a large effect in influencing provider price setting.
- A significant proportion of the variation in price is determined by cost variation, which suggests that hospitals have access to and make use of some cost information.
- Some limited empirical evidence for GPFH purchasers suggests that increased competition did reduce prices, especially for lower cost procedures and specialties. This may be because of more shopping around for these procedures and a greater willingness of patients to travel; because providers who are constrained from making losses are more comfortable discounting on lower cost procedures where discounts will be less visible; or because price-cost margins (and therefore scope for discounting) are greater for lower cost procedures.
- Competition appears to have a significant but delayed effect on costs.

✎ Activity 9.3

1 Summarize the theoretical effects of market competition. What are the main reasons why some have questioned the link between competition and price?

2 Link Propper and Soderlund's points about the market prerequisites for price competition in the NHS to the material in Chapter 8 on models of provider behaviour. What sorts of institutional arrangements are necessary for competitive forces to influence hospital behaviour?

3 What sorts of studies might you undertake to analyse the relationship between competition and prices? What are the main challenges to measuring the key variables of interest (market competition, price)?

Feedback

1 Market competition is supposed to force providers to reduce their prices (and in the longer term their costs) in order to attract business. According to this model, prices should be lower in markets where there is more competition (i.e. markets which are less concentrated). In practice, this relationship might not be observed in posted prices, since negotiations are private and may be reflected in actual prices paid (which are harder to measure empirically); providers and purchasers might need to engage in longer term relationships where price competition is not the main form of interaction; different services might be exposed to different degrees of competition; and the degree to which there is potential for price negotiation might depend on the degree of spare capacity that providers have. Competition could also manifest itself in competition on the basis of quality of care rather than price competition, particularly if purchasers do not face a hard budget constraint.

2 Competition is likely to influence provider behaviour only if managers are motivated to engage in this form of competition: this requires arrangements in which payment or reimbursement is in proportion to the number of patients seen (i.e. under a case-based payment system, or where patients pay user fees directly); and that managers' utility functions include some elements related to the size/prestige/surplus generated.

3 Cross-sectional studies of competition and price require measures of both variables. These must be available for a relatively large number of different markets where there is variation in each. Prices need to reflect the actual prices paid (rather than posted or list prices) and must be standardized to a particular product. Markets must be defined in terms of both geographical and product boundaries, and then concentration measures such as the n-firm concentration ratio or the HHI can be calculated.

Summary

You have learned about consumer behaviour in the health care market and how far patients are willing to behave like consumers in their interaction with the health care sector. You have also looked at ways of measuring the opportunity for competition between different health care providers. The theory relating competition to firm behaviour such as pricing was described and some of the shortcomings of this theory when applied to health care markets, particularly in predominantly public systems, were discussed.

References

Chalkey M and Malcolmson JM (1995) Contracts and competition in the NHS. Discussion Papers in Economics and Econometrics No. 9513. Southampton: University of Southampton, Department of Economics.

Dawson D (1994) Costs and prices in the internal market: Markets vs. the NHS Management Executive Guidelines. Centre for Health Economics Discussion Paper 115. York: Centre for Health Economics.

Donaldson C, Lloyd P and Lupton D (1991) Primary health care consumerism amongst elderly Australians. *Age and Ageing* 20(4): 280–6.

Hibbard JH and Weeks EC (1987) Consumerism in health care – prevalence and predictors. *Medical Care* 25(11): 1019–32.

Higgins J and Wiles R (1992) Study of patients who chose private health care for treatment. *British Journal of General Practice* 42(361): 326–9.

Lupton D (1997) Consumerism, reflexivity and the medical encounter. *Social Science & Medicine* 45: 373–81.

Lupton D, Donaldson C and Lloyd P (1991) Caveat-emptor or blissful ignorance – patients and the consumerist ethos. *Social Science & Medicine* 33: 559–68.

Nakamba P, Hanson K and McPake B (2002) Markets for hospital services in Zambia. *International Journal of Health Planning and Management* 17: 229–47.

Propper C and Soderlund N (1998) Competition in the NHS internal market: an overview of its effects on hospital prices and costs. *Health Economics* 7: 187–97.

Alternative models of provider competition

Overview

Traditional economic theories of competition predict that as the concentration of a market declines and competition becomes more intense, prices should fall. However, there is evidence from health care markets that this relationship does not always hold: in some contexts increased competition between hospitals has been associated with increased prices. For doctor service markets, it has been observed that increased competition is correlated with increased prices or utilization rates, leading to the hypothesis that doctors are able to induce demand. These findings have led to the questioning of the conventional economic wisdom and even whether the usual economic theory applies to health care markets. In this chapter you will review some of this evidence and the theoretical models that have been developed to accommodate these empirical observations. You will begin by looking at markets for medical services and then turn to markets for hospital services and insurance.

Learning objectives

By the end of this chapter you should be able to:

- describe how to measure the degree of concentration in health care markets
- discuss alternative models of medical behaviour and the evidence relating to supplier-induced demand
- describe the different forms that competition among hospitals can take
- understand the issue of risk selection by insurers.

Key terms

Monopolistic competition A market model which combines elements of monopoly (a downward-sloping demand curve) with competition (many sellers).

Purchaser-driven competition Market models in which the drive to shop around for superior price–quality combinations is dominated by institutional purchasers (health maintenance organizations or insurers).

Reputation goods Goods in which quality can only be judged by consumers through experience.

Risk selection The behaviour of insurers or providers who try to avoid patients with a higher than average risk of illness.

Supplier-induced demand Increased demand as a result of a provider (e.g. a doctor) exploiting an asymmetry of information.

Target income Part of the supplier-induced demand model which postulates that demand inducement is geared to the achievement of some target level of income.

Markets for medical (doctors') services

In considering the different market models earlier, you learned about the contrast between perfect competition and monopoly. Some of the characteristics of each of these two extremes are combined in the model of monopolistic competition, which is widely used to characterize markets for doctors' services. In monopolistic competition, the demand curve facing an individual provider slopes downwards, as in a monopoly, but there is an element of competition in the sense that there are a large number of sellers and firms ignore strategic interactions (Dranove and Satterthwaite 2000). Different doctors are imperfect substitutes for one another because of factors related to location, specialty, quality, individual patient preferences (implying a degree of product differentiation among providers) and possibly information imperfections (people are not aware of substitutes). Although interactions between providers are not strategic as in many oligopoly models, the downward-sloping demand curve means that a rise in price for one provider affects demand for others, though because of information or differentiation factors it will not completely eliminate demand for their services, as in the case of a perfectly competitive provider who faces a horizontal demand curve (Figure 10.1).

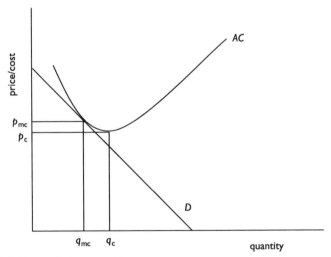

Figure 10.1 Monopolistic competition

Source: Phelps (2003)

Search costs and the increasing monopoly model

One model of medical markets considers the role of consumer information and search costs, and examines how an increase in the supply of doctors could lead to higher, not lower, prices. In this model, health services are modelled as reputation goods which have the following characteristics:

- They are differentiated from each other.
- Product quality is consumer-specific: individuals have idiosyncratic quality assessments of providers because they perceive attributes differently (e.g. they might have preferences over particular practice styles).
- The quality of a doctor's service can only be evaluated through the experience of actually using it.
- The product is sufficiently important to consumers that they will exert effort to find the seller with the price–quality combination that best suits them. This means that they will actively search, and this search process takes the form of asking for recommendations from friends and associates.

The model predicts that an increased supply of doctors can lead to an increase in prices. This happens because of two linked phenomena. First, the more doctors there are in a given community, the more difficulty consumers will have in finding a doctor of desired quality since this can only be determined through experience. Second, the more difficult the search, the less price-sensitive consumers become (Pauly and Satterthwaite 1981).

The predictions of the model come from some very specific assumptions about the type of questions people ask. Think about how the information yielded would differ if, instead of asking 'Do you know anything about Dr Smith?', you asked 'Can you recommend a good doctor?'. It is also important here to distinguish different types of care: the model might better describe the search for a primary care doctor than for a specialist, where a doctor's recommendation or referral might be a more important source of information.

Supplier-induced demand

You touched upon supplier-induced demand in Chapter 4. Here you will learn about the difficulties of empirically testing for such behaviour and the impact it may have on competition. Traditional views of supplier-induced demand include the following:

A bed built is a bed filled. (Roemer 1961)

Everyone knows that physicians exert a strong influence over the quantity and pattern of medical care demanded in a developed economy. (Evans 1974)

A 10% increase in the number of physicians is associated with a 3% increase in the rate of surgery. (Fuchs 1978)

The model of supplier-induced demand, in which providers respond to falling incomes (either because of some externally generated decrease in demand or reduction in prices) by shifting demand outwards to compensate, has been hotly debated by economists. The idea that demand is not exogenously given by consumer preferences and incomes is, however, problematic to economists who use demand curves to measure consumer welfare. One set of responses has been to show that the observed correlation between supply and utilization is also consistent with standard economic theory in which increased utilization may simply reflect a movement along a given demand curve when supply shifts outwards and prices fall; or that an increase in supply can reduce time and travel costs, leading to the same demand response.

Whether or not suppliers are actually able to induce demand is important because of a number of implications:

- Supply-side incentives, such as price controls, will not reduce expenditure if providers can compensate by increasing utilization.
- If demand is not determined exclusively by patients' own preferences but can be manipulated by the doctor in their agency role, then it is difficult to argue that demand curves reflect willingness to pay and can be used to measure consumer welfare.
- It raises the issue of whether health care markets can be analysed using the same economic tools as markets for other goods and services.

One reason why the debate has continued for so long is the difficulty of undertaking appropriate empirical testing of the model. Where testing is done using cross-sectional data on different markets where supply (market competition) varies, it is hard to distinguish whether high levels of supply are correlated with some unobserved variable which affects demand (e.g. income or a taste for medical procedures), and therefore higher supply is simply a response to higher demand; or whether higher supply has generated its own demand.

Theories have also had to propose factors which would act as limits to inducement behaviour by doctors. One explanation is in terms of target income, where doctors set their prices (if these are not controlled by an institutional purchaser) or quantities (through their agency role) to achieve a target income. Another is that doctors dislike inducing demand and they incur a psychic cost from behaving in a way which they perceive as being against the interests of their patients.

Empirical evidence in favour of the inducement hypothesis can be found in two papers. Gruber and Owings (1996) use the decline in fertility rates in the period 1970–82 in the USA as a shock to obstetrician incomes. They find that in the states where fertility fell the most, the Caesarian section rate (for which doctors received higher average reimbursement than for a normal delivery) increased most. Yip (1998) found that thoracic surgeons were able to compensate for a reduction in incomes due to a decline in Medicare reimbursement rates for coronary by-pass grafting by increasing the volume and intensity of procedures. Other evidence has found a relationship between referrals for medical tests and doctors' ownership of diagnostic laboratories (Hillman *et al.* 1990, 1992).

The weight of evidence seems to lie in favour of there being a degree of inducement by doctors. However, there are alternative models, such as the search model described above, that yield similar predictions about the relationship between supply and price which do not require the assumption of inducement. It is important also to make the link between doctors' behaviour and the way they are organized and paid: inducement requires there to be a financial reward to encouraging additional services which does not arise under salary and capitation payment. In some payment systems, such as capitation, there is a risk that doctors under-provide and skimp on care (supplier-discouraged demand). Perhaps the most important lesson from this literature is that doctors respond to financial incentives in ways that have both clinical and economic consequences.

Competition in markets for hospital services

Health sector reforms in many parts of the world have incorporated structural changes that encourage competition between hospitals. These include the splitting of purchasers and providers, measures to increase hospital autonomy and increased reliance on payments from patients. The aims of such reforms are usually some combination of increasing efficiency (reducing costs) and improving quality. But what evidence is there of the effects of hospital competition?

Quality competition and the medical arms race: USA and Thailand

There are a number of reasons why the standard economic model of price competition may not apply in the market for health services. First, the presence of third party purchasers such as insurers undermines consumer sensitivity to price. Second, non-profit organizations are important providers in many health care markets, particularly hospitals. The behaviour of such providers may be better explained by managerial models where hospital managers pursue quality rather than profit (see Chapter 8), or by behaviour to attract doctors who then attract patients. Third, health services are not homogeneous products: their quality varies in complex ways and shopping around for the right price–quality combination may be difficult for relatively uninformed consumers.

In such markets, competition among providers may be based on quality. This model suggests that providers respond to more competition (lower concentration) not by dropping prices but by increasing quality. These quality improvements are often (but not always) associated with greater investment in high technology equipment and the hotel aspects of care. Hospitals attempt to signal their quality through characteristics which are more readily observed by poorly informed patients. Another reason for investing in equipment and facilities is for hospitals to attract doctors, and thereby their patients. Analysts have attributed the medical arms race which saw dramatic increases in hospital costs in the USA through to the early 1980s to these factors. Thailand saw an explosion in the availability of high-tech facilities in private hospitals in the 1990s. The following edited extract from Nittayaramphong and Tangcharoensathien (1994) examines trends in private sector provision in Thailand.

📖 Private sector provision in Thailand

The number of doctors working in the private sector has steadily increased over the years . . . Many public physicians work out-of-hours in the private sector to supplement their income. Despite the long hours worked by MOPH [Ministry of Public Health] doctors, their total income is still considerably lower than those who work much shorter hours, but full time, in the private sector.

The rapidly changing picture of MOPH manpower can be explained in terms of both 'push and pull'. Rapid private growth and the income differential between the public and private sectors serve to pull both doctors and nurses into the private sector. In public hospitals, doctors' workloads are much higher and remuneration levels similar to those of teachers and other civil servants, pushing doctors out of the public sector.

So far there has been a piecemeal approach to the problem, but giving minute incentives to health professionals will not halt the brain drain. Currently, the major obstacle is posed by the Ministry of Finance which will not allow public hospitals to use their revenue flexibly. If hospital revenues could be used to provide incentive payments to professionals then the brain drain may be decreased . . .

The MOPH is particularly concerned about the equity implications of the growth of the private sector; it is anxious that a two-tier health care system providing private care for the wealthy and public services for the poor does not develop . . .

In addition to hospital and clinic facilities in Thailand, private providers of special diagnostic services have recently become widespread. In particular, private sector use of computerized tomographic (CT) scanners, magnetic resonance imaging (MRI) and extracorporeal shock wave lithotripters (ESWL) has grown rapidly recently and has become a matter of serious concern.

Non-price competition between private hospitals contributes to the procurement of high cost medical technologies such as CT scanners . . . A ratio of 10 scanners per million population in Bangkok reflects a bizarre health care system. There is no effective mechanism to oversee and control the procurement and distribution of medical technologies. On the contrary, the government indirectly promotes the accumulation of high technology equipment. This occurs in two ways. The Board of Investment exempts import duties for medical equipment for registered health care companies and the Ministry of Finance has a customs policy whereby all X-ray equipment used in medicine has been totally duty-exempt since 1988.

The race is now on to procure other high technology equipment such as ESWLs and MRIs. As of June 1991 there were a total of five MRI machines in Thailand, all of which were owned and operated by the private sector. Public sector facilities are trying to procure machines, but funding for these items is limited. At the same date there were 16 ESWLs in Thailand; although eleven were sited in public hospitals, some of these were owned and operated by the private sector. An evaluation of this 'contracting in' of high technology equipment is planned . . .

Private hospital growth is a result of increasing demand for private care amongst the better off and excess demand at public hospitals. However, the Board of Investment has also played a significant role stimulating the boom through corporate tax and customs duty exemption for private hospital construction. The Ministry of Finance customs duty policy in 1988 to exempt X-ray machines from duty and non-price competition have stimulated the accumulation of high cost medical technologies. Evidence shows abuses of these machines which raise health care costs and encourage inefficiency.

Policy should address the integration of the private health sector into a national health development plan through closer collaboration and policy dialogue. Two of the most urgent issues are: first, the oversupply of private beds in Bangkok; and second, the severe brain drain situation. Policies on private hospital investment should be shifted to the regional level.

Efforts should be made to control the procurement and distribution of high cost technologies and their use. Financing mechanisms seem to have high potential to control cost escalation. The Civil Servant Medical Benefit Scheme should be developed to be more efficient and not to aggravate inequity.

 Activity 10.1

1 The health care system was characterized by a boom in private hospital provision, encouraged by increased demand for private care facilities and by favourable tax and customs duty exemptions. What implications did this increased supply have for the market?
2 How did these facilities attract customers and which customers did they attract?
3 What impact did the expanding private sector have on the public sector?

 Feedback

1 The increased supply of private facilities has led to market concentration, particularly in urban areas.

2 Hospitals are using non-price competition mechanisms to attract consumers, mainly through the provision of new facilities and by offering high-cost medical technologies. There are issues about the appropriateness of the use of this technology in some cases. It is mainly the wealthier sector of the population who are able to afford and use these services.

3 The public sector is being affected by a brain drain of doctors and other personnel who are attracted by the higher wages offered in the private sector. With wealthier patients seeking their treatment in the private sector, this may have a negative impact on public sector activities in terms of the types and quality of services provided, potentially creating a two-tier system of health care.

Quality, informed purchasers and payer-driven competition

One reason why patients rely on structural signs of quality, such as equipment and amenities, is that they are usually unable to assess quality of care, in particular the health outcomes.

Two developments offer the possibility of increasing attention paid to quality of care and, potentially, to the effect of competition on quality. The first is increased production of publicly available performance reports. Hospital report cards, which include measures of health outcomes, have been produced in the USA, Canada and the UK. Such data are thought to encourage competition among providers on outcomes, rather than merely structural, aspects of quality.

Activity 10.2

What risks are posed by the provision of information to the public on the clinical outcomes of care provided by facilities or individual doctors?

 Feedback

While such improvements in public information about clinical quality are to be welcomed, there are two risks. The first is that providers might turn away the more complicated cases in order to maintain their quality score if case mix is not taken into account. The other is that information about provider outcomes may only influence those facilities that face effective competition: in smaller markets, patients may not have any choice but to visit the lower quality providers.

A second development in health care markets is the shift from patient-driven to purchaser-driven competition (Dranove and Satterthwaite 2000). This is best exemplified in the USA where, in managed care, purchasers contract selectively with providers and have an incentive to seek the best value for services; at the same time they are able more effectively to process information on clinical outcomes and use this to market their plans to the public. The increased role of informed purchasers in the health care market can also be seen in the purchasing relationships embodied in primary organizations in the UK which purchase services from providers on the behalf of specified populations; and purchasing relationships between the ministry of health and providers (governmental and/or non-governmental) in, for example, Zambia and Uganda.

The effect of purchaser-driven competition: the experience of the US health system

Health maintenance organizations (HMOs) and preferred provider organizations (PPOs) – as opposed to a fee-for-service (FFS) system – are managed care plans where coverage is paid in advance.

- An HMO is a service delivery system that provides coverage for hospital and physician services for a prepaid fixed fee. HMO members choose from among providers that have been contracted by the organization.
- A PPO is a health care arrangement that offers incentives to use health care providers within the network of the organization. PPO members can save on deductibles and co-payments if they use providers contracted by the organization.

McPake *et al.* (2002) found, from a review of the literature, evidence that there is an increasing impact of managed care on prices. This trend towards price competition under the influence of managed care arrangements has also been shown in a large sample of US hospitals.

In their study of price competition and hospital cost growth in the United States, Bemazai *et al.* (1999) demonstrated that, with the rapid spread of HMOs and PPOs, health care costs in the USA slowed down. The authors used regression analysis to study the association between hospital operating costs and a range of key independent variables such as the penetration of an area with managed care organizations, and the number of competitors as measured by the HHI (see Chapter 9). The following extract highlights some salient points.

 Effects of managed care on prices

Our results suggest that managed care's effects, first observed in California, are now spreading throughout the US. In other words, managed care's expansion in the US is changing the underlying market dynamic by placing greater importance on price competition instead of the traditional quality and service-based (non-price) competition.

Hospitals in high managed care penetration areas (that is, areas with high HMO or high PPO penetration) displayed a significantly lower rate of cost growth between 1989 and 1994. Our findings, however, also suggest that the ability of managed care plans to slow hospital cost growth is critically dependent upon the level of hospital competition. The estimated managed care effect – that is, the difference in hospital cost growth between high and low managed care penetration areas – is statistically significant only in the case of hospitals located in highly competitive hospital markets.

This study also provides preliminary empirical evidence on the relative effectiveness of HMOs compared to PPOs in controlling hospital cost growth. It has been hypothesized that HMOs exercise greater cost control relative to PPOs for several reasons. First, HMOs typically construct more restrictive provider networks endowing the HMO with greater leverage in negotiating contracts with health care providers. Second, some HMOs pay physicians and hospitals on a capitated basis while PPOs rely almost exclusively on price discounts. Capitation endows physicians with stronger incentives to reduce hospital costs than discounted fees. Our study, although unable to separate the independent effects of alternative payment mechanisms, does provide an aggregate estimate of the relative effect of HMO versus PPO penetration on hospital cost growth. For example, at a theoretical limiting case of HHI equal to zero (highly competitive markets), hospital cost growth was 15.3% less in high HMO penetration areas compared to medium or low HMO penetration areas, and 7.7% less in high PPO penetration areas compared to medium or low PPO penetration areas.

 Activity 10.3

1 Does price or quality competition prevail in the USA?
2 Do you think price competition is beneficial to consumers?
3 Can you think of any examples of price competition in your own country's health care markets?

 Feedback

1 Bamezai *et al.* (1999) report that managed care in the USA is placing greater importance on price competition. The effects of price competition in relation to minimizing cost growth is reported to be dependent on the level of hospital competition and managed care penetration levels in an area. HMOs were reported to be more effective

than PPOs in containing costs through the mechanisms of restricting provider networks and maintaining tighter contract control over providers and per-capita reimbursement of doctors and hospitals in some areas.

2 The experience is mixed. As the example shows, price competition can bring health care costs down, but it can also have detrimental effects on consumers because providers may reduce quality or try to cut corners. In response to this, many US states have passed laws to regulate managed care markets in order to improve consumer protection.

3 You may find examples of price competition in parts of the health care sector in many countries – for example, private practitioner fees, insurance markets or over-the-counter drug markets.

Competition among purchasers and risk selection

Another part of the health care market is made up of purchasers, who may also be competing for patients. While competition might be expected to increase the choice available to consumers as well as to reduce prices, health policy makers and researchers have focused on risk selection as a possible outcome with negative effects. Risk selection takes place when economic agents in a health system take advantage of unpriced differences in risk among individuals to break risk pooling arrangements in order to increase profits. This can take place in the context of risk pooling because payment is based on average expected cost, and opportunities exist to preferentially attract those who are likely to incur costs less than the average. Risk selection is sometimes called cream skimming and is most likely to take place under some form of prospective payment system (e.g. in the case of insurance premia or payment through capitation systems). Health reforms that encourage competition between prospectively paid providers (e.g. GPs paid by capitation) or health plans/insurers may lead to greater incentives for risk selection. Risk selection is closely related to adverse selection. The following excerpt from Puig-Junoy (1999) describes risk selection in health insurance.

📖 Managing risk selection

Risk selection in the health insurance and the health care markets, as an undesirable outcome of unpriced risk heterogeneity, may take several forms. Given a fixed prospective price paid to the firms for a heterogeneous product, they may select 'good' risks on the basis of enrollees, patients, services and quality (i.e. how much treatment is provided). Risk selection increases transaction costs as a result of the efforts to attract good risks. Risk selection also introduces the possibility of under-provision of services . . . unless countervailing forces check this tendency. Both trends represent the efficiency cost of risk selection.

Uniformity of pricing for heterogeneous groups of services appears as inherently related to health care markets. Price or reimbursement regulation is at the root of the problem. Equity requires community rated or income related premiums (cross-subsidies between risk groups) in the insurance market. Premiums are regulated to prevent risk rating in order to keep premiums affordable for high risk and low income groups. Consequently, incentives to exploit unpriced risk heterogeneity are stronger under competitive pressures than under traditional retrospective reimbursement methods.

The existence of asymmetric and imperfect information in the agency relationship between insured and insurer and between purchaser and provider is at the root of the risk selection problem. Selection incentives would be minimized if insurers and providers were reimbursed at the exact patient cost. A uniform fully prospective payment for a heterogeneous group of persons gives insurers and providers the maximum incentive to compete in wasteful ways to select good risks and avoid bad ones. The more insurers and providers are exposed to competition, the greater will be their efforts to attract good financial risks. Thus, providing that there is no market power, risk selection should be the main reason for regulating or limiting the role of competition.

 Activity 10.4

   1   What factors encourage risk selection by insurers?
   2   What are the consequences of risk selection by insurers?
   3   Are there any opportunities for risk selection (either by purchasers or providers) in your system?

 Feedback

1 Risk selection is encouraged when there is competition because successful risk selection can increase profits. Uniform payments also encourage risk selection because this creates an opportunity to earn profits by identifying those who are at lower than average risk.

2 Equity is affected as the pooling of risks between healthier and sicker individuals is undermined; this leads to ever-increasing insurance premia for those at higher risk. Risk selection also creates inefficiencies through increased transactions costs associated with efforts to attract good risks. There is the possibility of undertreatment.

3 Risk selection can emerge from competing insurers, or even when provider payment systems do not recognize heterogeneity of costs between patients (for instance, in diagnostic related group systems, hospitals may try to select against high cost patients, or primary care doctors paid through a capitation system may try to avoid costly patients such as the elderly).

Summary

You have examined the different models which have been developed to explain the effects of competition among providers (doctors, hospitals) and purchasers (e.g. insurers). You have seen that competition in the health sector can have quite different effects from those predicted under standard economic theory. These can influence both efficiency and equity.

References

Bemazai A, Zwanziger J, Melnick GA and Mann JM (1999) Price competition and hospital cost growth in the United States (1989–1994). *Health Economics* 8: 233–43.

Dranove D and Satterthwaite MA (2000) The industrial organization of health care markets, in Culyer AJ and Newhouse JP (eds) *Handbook of Health Economics*, Vol. 1A. Amsterdam: North-Holland.

Evans RG (1974) Supplier-induced demand: some empirical evidence and implications, in Perlman M (ed) *The Economics of Health and Medical Care*. London: Macmillan.

Fuchs V (1978) The supply of surgeons and the demand for operations. *Journal of Human Resources* 13 (Supplement): 35–56.

Gruber J and Owings M (1996) Physician financial incentives and cesarean section delivery. *RAND Journal of Economics* 27: 99–123.

Hillman BJ, Joseph CA, Mabry MR, Sunshine JH, Kennedy SD and Noether M (1990) Frequency and costs of diagnostic imaging in office practice – a comparison of self-referring and radiologist-referring physicians. *New England Journal of Medicine* 323: 1604–8.

Hillman BJ, Olson GT, Griffith PE, Sunshine JH, Joseph CA, Kennedy SD, Nelson WR and Bernhardt LB (1992) Physicians' utilization and charges for outpatient diagnostic imaging in a Medicare population. *Journal of the American Medical Association* 268: 2050–4.

McPake B, Kumaranayake L and Normand C (2002) *Health Economics: An International Perspective*. London: Routledge.

Nittayaramphong A and Tangcharoensathien V (1994) Thailand: private health care out of control? *Health Policy and Planning* 9(1): 31–40.

Pauly MV and Satterthwaite MA (1981) The pricing of primary care physicians services: a test of the role of consumer information. *Bell Journal of Economics* 12(2): 488–506.

Phelps CE (2003) *Health Economics*, 3rd edn. Reading, MA: Addison-Wesley.

Puig-Junoy J (1999) Managing risk selection incentives in health sector reforms. *International Journal of Health Planning and Management* 14: 287–311.

Roemer MI (1961) Bed supply and hospital utilization: a natural experiment. *Hospitals, the Journal of the American Hospital Association* 35: 36–42.

Yip W (1998) Physician responses to medical fee reductions: changes in the volume and intensity of supply of coronary artery bypass graft (CABG) surgeries in the medicare and private sectors. *Journal of Health Economics* 17: 675–700.

11 The economic rationale for government involvement in the health sector

Overview

Although the past two decades have seen an international trend towards promoting private sector activity, government involvement in health care delivery remains substantial in most countries. In general, public spending accounts for a substantial portion of all health care spending; governments are deeply involved in producing as well as financing health care services and they play a role in the structuring of relationships with the private sector through the use of regulation and contracting.

This chapter discusses the rationale for government involvement in the health sector. It initially examines the notion of market failure and then goes on to discuss regulation as one of the main avenues for such involvement.

Learning objectives

After working through this chapter you should be able to:

- describe the rationale for government involvement in the health sector
- outline the competition versus regulation debate
- outline the reasons for regulation in the health sector.

Key terms

Adverse selection When a party enters into an agreement in which they can use their own private information to the disadvantage of another party.

Externality Cost or benefit arising from an individual's production or consumption decision which indirectly affects the well-being of others.

Moral hazard A situation in which one of the parties to an agreement has an incentive, after the agreement is made, to act in a manner that brings additional benefits to themselves at the expense of the other party.

Theory of the second best Theory providing the economic rationale for government intervention in situations of market failure.

Government involvement in the health sector and market failure

It is conventionally argued that government involvement in the economy is justified when there is a failure of markets to achieve the most efficient outcomes through competition. One of the problems with this line of argument, however, is that it assumes that, in an ideal world, markets are somehow independent of government intervention. Government involvement, however, is generally crucial to the proper functioning of markets – in particular, in establishing the right institutional conditions through creating the appropriate rules for the various actors in the marketplace. For instance, this extends to maintaining a system of property rights and ensuring that they are properly enforced. This point is worth remembering particularly when you later consider the regulation versus competition debate. For now, you will examine the issue of market failure more closely and highlight some of the reasons for it. There are six reasons to consider.

Monopoly power

Firms with monopoly power will maximize profits by restricting output, thereby charging a price that is greater than that which would emerge in competitive markets (i.e. closer to marginal cost). This gap, representing the loss of utility to those consumers priced out of the market, creates a welfare loss and is inefficient.

Externalities

Externalities occur when the private costs or benefits associated with the consumption of a good or service exceed the costs or benefits to the individual consumer. In other words, there is a spillover of costs or benefits that may not be accounted for in an individual's consumption decision. An example is a factory that pollutes, creating a negative externality because it imposes a cost on society over and above the cost of production incurred by the owners. Thus markets where this form of production is uncontrolled will have a tendency to encourage overpollution. Another example, relevant to health, is vaccination and the positive externality an individual receiving vaccination confers on the wider community in terms of promoting herd immunity.

Common property resources

These are resources that are owned by no one person and may be used by many. The classic example is that of the world's international fishing grounds and the problem of overfishing. Efforts to conserve fish stocks through quotas or some form of restriction are only feasible if they are universally adhered to. The problem with achieving this is that each participant is unlikely to voluntarily cut back on their catch since there is no guarantee that others will do likewise – indeed, by voluntarily cutting back he/she is effectively increasing the amount available to those who do not cooperate. With common property resources, the failure to achieve such cooperation means that the level of activity in general will tend to be higher than is socially optimal (which in principle is the level of output that would occur if each fisherman bore the full cost of his/her catch; the full cost would include the conservation value of each fish). Such incentives structures are often referred to as *the prisoners' dilemma* (as you learned in Chapter 7) or *the collective action problem* where cooperative solutions among self-interested parties are stymied by the problem that in order to cooperate, each individual becomes open to the possibility of exploitation by others. In these instances, the argument for government regulation is that it imposes a socially optimal solution that may not otherwise be achieved through voluntary cooperation.

Public goods

These are goods whose total cost of production does not increase as the number of consumers increases. The two key characteristics of public goods are that they are non-rival (the amount that one person consumes should not affect the amount that other people consume, e.g. a street-light) and non-excludable (once this good is produced there is no way to stop anyone else from consuming it, e.g. the creation of an army for national defence will protect everyone).

In the case of a pure public good, these characteristics will mean that people will not be willing to pay for something that they could get if someone else bought the good. Thus there would be no private market for a pure public good. In practice, the degree of non-rivalness and non-excludability will vary, and since it is difficult to charge users to cover the costs of production, the private market will produce an output lower than the socially efficient level of output. This again represents an example of the collective action problem, but this time in reverse to the previous example (as it encourages under- rather than overproduction). In this instance, individuals who do not contribute to the cost of a public good are nonetheless able to free-ride on the contributions of those who do.

Asymmetric information

The presence of perfect information is one of the key assumptions in a perfectly competitive economy. In some cases information occurs as a public good (e.g. once the information is known to anyone it is often easily available to others). Two important sources of failure when privately held information is bought or sold are *adverse selection* and *moral hazard*. An example of adverse selection occurs when individuals are able to conceal information regarding their risk of ill health when purchasing insurance. An example of moral hazard occurs when individuals alter their behaviour by taking greater health risks once they have purchased health insurance.

Missing markets

Another reason for market inefficiency is that the market for a certain good may simply not exist. An example is the case of the pure public good. Another important set of missing markets is related to insurance. Insured risks need to be independent and for this reason it is not possible to insure for the consequences of warfare or natural disasters where large populations are at risk and where individuals' risks are correlated. For example, it is difficult to insure crops against bad weather because all the farmers in a given locality have the same probability of suffering from the same bad weather and an insurance company may have to compensate them all. Insurance works by pooling independent risks. Health insurance is based on the assumption that only a certain proportion of clients will be affected by illness in any one year, and therefore when risks are not independent, as when there is a major epidemic, risk pooling is not possible.

Where markets fail for any of these reasons, government has a range of options to intervene – for example, through regulation of insurance markets or by providing public health services which would not otherwise be efficiently allocated by markets.

 Activity 11.1

Think about the above reasons for market failure and note down examples from your experience in health services. What interventions could governments choose to overcome the adverse outcomes of markets in these areas?

 Feedback

The sorts of examples you may have thought of include the following:

- There may be only one hospital in a small market (monopoly power).
- If individuals paid privately for all immunizations they would not take into account the social benefit of lowering the prevalence rate of different diseases (externalities).
- No one would buy most preventive measures such as public information campaigns (a public good).
- Where private insurance markets are missing, for example in disaster relief, government needs to step in (missing markets).

Failure of markets to achieve social goals

In addition to issues of market failure and consequently the failure of markets to allocate resources efficiently, markets may also be seen to be inappropriate because they do not achieve other social goals – notably equity. Some of the equity arguments that could be posited in opposition to the presence of markets are as follows.

Caring externality

This idea is based on the observation that individuals seem to derive a positive externality from the consumption of health care by others. It seems to derive from the concern that individuals have that others receive (or at least have access to) treatment when it is needed. This characteristic of health care seems to set it apart from other goods and services – for example, it is difficult to see how such a caring externality would apply to the consumption of motor vehicles, restaurant meals, tickets to the football and so on. This is discussed further in Chapter 17.

Distributional considerations

An important characteristic of the market economy is that it allocates goods and services on the basis of individuals' willingness and ability to pay for them. In health care this can mean that certain groups are excluded from access to needed services.

Protecting individuals from others

Profit- or revenue-maximizing behaviour may lead to exploitation of individuals in ways that society finds offensive (e.g. child labour or hazardous working conditions).

Merit goods

These are goods that society deems to be especially important (such as education and health care) and society may feel individuals should be required or encouraged to consume. Thus, even if the price system allocates goods and services with complete efficiency, members of society may not want to rely solely on the market since it may deny individuals access to these merit goods.

 Activity 11.2

How are these social goals reflected in your country's health system?

 Feedback

You may have identified a range of redistribution policies relating to financing and provision of health care in your country. Examples of protecting consumers from profit-maximizing behaviour include subsidizing drug prices and capping provider fees. Depending on their cultural and historical background, many societies would see health care as a merit good. But there is an ongoing debate about the trade-offs between achieving efficiency and equity, and the sequencing of these goals (Cullis and Jones 1992). While some societies have enacted access to health care as a basic right in their laws, others would see this as paternalistic.

The theory of the second best

The *theory of the second best* is directed towards the question of government policy formulation in an economy in which there is market failure. It is concerned with the correction of market failure and the achievement of what would be regarded as a desirable distribution of income.

Economic theory posits that a perfectly competitive economy will yield the 'first best', that is, a resource allocation which cannot be improved upon in the Pareto-optimal sense. The theory of the second best suggests that if the first best outcome is not obtained due to the presence of a distortion (e.g. leading to market failure), then the next best outcome from a policy maker's viewpoint will be the introduction of another 'distortion' (i.e. government action). Government action can take many forms – regulation being one. The standard 'tools' for such action include:

- rules and regulations
- public ownership/provision of goods
- government expenditure (financing)
- taxation.

The competition versus regulation debate

There has long been a competition versus regulation debate within the health sector. However, you should note that these concepts are not mutually exclusive. Forms of competition can take place in a highly regulated environment and elements of regulation can be present in highly competitive markets. It is important to recognize that competition generally requires certain ground rules and that such rules often come in the form of regulation. An example of this relationship between regulation and competition might be seen in the pharmaceutical market where certain regulations ensuring a degree of consumer safety are needed for competitive markets to emerge.

Those who advocate less regulation by government over the private sector tend to do so by arguing that this promotes greater competition. Where they see a role for the state in influencing the activities of the private sector, such advocates tend to then favour the use of financial incentives over direct regulatory control.

In contrast, regulation proponents call for a greater role for the state in the delivery and regulation of health care. Furthermore, they argue that excessive reliance on competition in health care leads to problems of excessive accumulation of high technology equipment and inappropriate provision of certain services.

However, in many low- and middle-income countries the relevance of this debate over more or less regulation is diminished by the limitations on the capacity of governments to finance and provide services. Consequently, perhaps more by default, the private health sector in many of these countries forms a large component of health care. If regulation is seen as a means to discourage perverse practices arising from market failures and to help address equity concerns, then the existence of effective regulatory capacity within the health sector can be considered crucial to the success of policies that encourage greater participation of the private sector and competition. In many low- and middle-income countries, however, the capacity of governments to regulate effectively cannot be assumed.

The following extract from a discussion paper from Lilani Kumaranayake (1998) describes the main reason for more private sector activity.

 Main reasons for the global increase in private sector activity

1. *A deliberate policy choice (e.g. health sector reform)*

Encouraging the development of the private sector as an alternative means of health care provision has been an explicit part of health sector reform packages. This has been spurred on by increasing resource constraints and the poor performance of the public sector. These scarce resources were often allocated inefficiently (e.g. towards curative rather than preventative care). Services were often of poor quality, with long waiting times and inadequate drugs/supplies ... The poor performance of the public sector, increasing economic difficulties and changes in prevailing ideologies led to calls for a reduction in the role of the state and an increased role for the private sector ... Through increasingly competitive markets for health care, privatisation has been seen as a way to improve resource allocation, efficiency and quality, as well as to broaden consumer choice:

- The private sector was seen as having fewer administrative and political constraints than public bureaucracies, thus improving the efficiency and effectiveness of health services.
- The introduction of competition was thought to lead to improvements in the quality of services and consumer satisfaction ... for example, private clinics in Bombay are open in the evenings with shorter waiting times and often have a ready supply of pharmaceuticals.
- Increased privatisation was thought to be a means to free up resources which could be allocated to the more needy in society – the idea behind this was that those consumers willing to pay for health care would now choose to use private sector services, freeing up public resources.
- Countries may initiate privatisation through the changing of existing laws and regula-tions. For example, Tanzania repealed its previous ban against private practice by health professionals and facilities. Professionals can now operate their own clinics and consult-ation rooms, and private pharmacies can now operate in competition with public ones. In addition to changing legislation, many countries have actively encouraged the development and expansion of the private sector. For example, in 1981 Chile promoted the creation of prepaid insurance schemes. These ISAPREs operated like health maintenance organisations .... To further encourage the ISAPREs, Chileans were even allowed to transfer their mandatory earnings contribution previously going to the state (about 4% of wages) to their selected ISAPRE plan.

2. *A response to weak provision of public health services and rapid increase in informal sector activity*

The development of private sector activity also emerged spontaneously, independently of the policy regime. Again in response to poor and inadequate public services, there has been a rapid development of informal private sector provision of health care. This can be characterized by individuals operating for profit. These providers are often untrained or unlicensed, but are seen as a source of inexpensive care by patients. These providers can range from health care professionals operating at home or other premises to the drug-seller on the street corner.

3. *Response to increased consumer affluence (e.g. increasing middle class) and preference for higher quality services*

Particularly in fast-growing economies of South-East Asia and Latin America, as well as urban areas in many low- and middle-income countries, the demand for private sector care has been driven by its being seen as a higher quality service. In this context, we no longer see just individual providers working alone, but now have the emergence of clinics/hospitals as well as private companies organising private health care (some of these companies are even listed on national stock exchanges). In areas where patients/consumers have increased demand for private care, we often see the use of high technology equipment.

 Activity 11.3

Do you think these reasons apply in your country?

 Feedback

You need to consider each of the following reasons:

- encouragement of private sector provision in recent health care reforms
- expansion in response to weaknesses of the public sector
- expansion in response to increased consumer affluence.

The introduction of competitive markets into health care provision, mainly through a policy of privatization, has been seen as a way to potentially improve resource allocation, efficiency and quality, and increased consumer choice and satisfaction. This is particularly the case when the government is experiencing economic difficulties. As mentioned previously, however, ultimately such reforms are political decisions and pivotal to these decisions are often the values and interests of key stakeholders.

Regulation and markets in health care

You have seen that markets sometimes fail or do not achieve certain social objectives such as equity. It is now worth turning more specifically to the nature and role of government in addressing these issues in health care. Government potentially has three levels of responsibility in the health sector: as a payer/purchaser, as a provider and as a regulator of health services. In practice, the roles governments generally take on range from the simple one of regulator – leaving financing and provision to the private sector – to the more significant one of bearing responsibility for both financing and provision of health care. That a society ascribes a greater role, for instance, to government as a regulator than as a provider of health services (and therefore a greater role for the private sector) is a decision that is determined in the political sphere through the interplay of the values and interests that are relevant to policy makers (Evans 1997).

Maynard (1982) identifies three concerns of regulation in relation to health services: prices, quality and quantity. A regulatory mechanism (or regulatory instrument) refers to the specific method used to affect these three factors. These regulatory mechanisms can be thought of in two ways:

- as legal controls – legislated requirements that can lead to punitive action if they are not met
- as incentives which can be used to affect (enable) price, quantity or quality.

The following abstract from an article by Maria Goddard (2003) discusses the areas of the health sector that provide scope for regulatory action. One point that she makes is that there has been a great deal of emphasis in recent years on using regulation to provide more information to consumers.

📖 Regulation of health care markets

Regulation can take many forms. Public ownership or provision is an extreme form of regulation where the market is replaced, thus protecting the consumer from potential exploitation at the hands of private providers operating in a market where they are not subjected to the discipline of competition. However, wholesale replacement of the market may not be the only (or best) answer to market failure. At the other end of the spectrum, the market can be tweaked in order to create the characteristics of the perfectly competitive situation . . . 'Market-displacing' and 'market-facilitating' strategies both offer a potential answer to market failure.

Regulation can tackle different aspects of the market. The structure–conduct–performance paradigm holds that a causal relationship exists between market structure (e.g. number of buyers and sellers), conduct of providers (e.g. price setting, decisions on quality) and economic performance in terms of efficiency and welfare. Regulation of *structure* has been a dominant force in many health care markets. In the US, anti-trust legislation is used extensively to regulate both horizontal and vertical mergers in health care. However, hospital markets have still become more concentrated and there has been a dramatic growth in multi-hospital systems, integrated delivery systems and joint ventures in the US. Overall, evidence about the impact on costs, prices and quality of more concentrated hospital markets tends to be inconclusive. Regulation of the conduct of organizations that hold market power is common – for example, in the utilities industries in the UK. The existence of natural monopoly (where it is only efficient to have one or a small number of providers in the market at one time) means regulation focuses on issues such as pricing and profit, quality standards and collusive behaviour. In health care markets, the likelihood of natural monopoly suggests that regulation of conduct will be appropriate. Indeed, in publicly funded systems, where extensive spare capacity and duplication of services are not desirable, the behaviour of monopoly providers is often curtailed through rules relating to pricing, profits, quality and access. The UK has probably been one of the most intensely regulated health care systems in this respect, although recent English NHS policy on 'foundation hospitals' is directed at reducing central regulation of selected public hospitals in return for good performance. In almost all health care systems, substantial regulation of the behaviour of professionals exists, both in the form of self-regulation and also through external standard setting and training requirements.

Asymmetry of information is one of the major causes of market failures in health care . . . Recent improvements in health information may have helped to mitigate this to some extent. Information may relate to inputs (e.g. availability of specialists, staff–patient ratios), processes (e.g. waiting times, length of stay), or outcomes (e.g. mortality and morbidity rates from treatment), and includes the wealth of information on health and health care appearing on the internet across the world, as well as comparative performance data on providers. In principle, such information reduces the gap in knowledge between buyers and sellers, strengthening the position of the buyer. In markets that are already characterized by some degree of supply-side competition, this may provide a better basis for making choices. If coupled with efforts to enhance the power of purchasers of care (as in the development of managed care in the US and the strengthening of the sickness funds in the Netherlands), the efficacy of this approach may be further increased. Even where choice of provider is more limited, improvements in the availability of comparative data can have an impact if they provide the impetus for providers to improve their performance. Such an approach can also work in systems with limited patient choice but strong government control over providers. In this situation, resource allocation or other rewards and sanctions can be based on comparative performance.

However, despite the explosion of such information, it appears to have had limited impact on improving performance. In the US, the emphasis has been on supplying comparative information on clinical performance in the form of report cards, provider profiles and consumer reports. The public appears to make little use of this information, although providers appear to take notice and may as a result adjust their behaviour, but not always in the desired direction – e.g. in the UK, the limited evidence on the use of such data suggests a modest impact on consumers, providers and purchasers.

 Activity 11.4

The author is sceptical as to the effectiveness of regulation. Why is that so?

 Feedback

The assumption underlying this type of regulation is that the failure of markets occurs due to a lack of information, and thus providing information is a sufficient condition for achieving desired social objectives. Such an assumption may overlook other important influences on the conduct of individuals such as incentives and power relations. For instance, providing patients with clinical performance information is likely to be of limited effectiveness in bringing about behaviour change if patients feel powerless to question the type of treatment or service they are offered.

Summary

You have examined the economic rationale for regulation and discussed the growing importance of the issues as health care systems become more market-oriented. Government involvement in the health sector is considered a vital element in these reforms and is used as a means to improve the functioning of markets, to address negative or perverse consequences of market behaviour/competition, and to ensure equity and access to services within the health sector.

References

Cullis J and Jones P (1992) *Public Finance and Public Choice: Analytical Perspectives*. London: McGraw-Hill.

Evans RG (1997) Going for the gold: the redistributive agenda behind market-based health care reform. *Journal of Health Politics, Policy and Law* 22(2): 427–65.

Goddard M (2003) Regulation of health care markets. *Journal of Health Services Research and Policy* 8(4): 193–5.

Kumaranayake L (1998) *Economic Aspects of Health Sector Regulation: Strategic Choices for Low and Middle Income Countries*. Public Health Policy Departmental Publication 29, London School of Hygiene & Tropical Medicine.

Maynard A (1982) The regulation of public and private health care markets, in McLachlan G and Maynard A (eds) *A Public/Private Mix for Health: The Relevance and Effects of Change*. London: Nuffield Provincial Hospitals Trust.

12 Economic theories of regulation

Overview

This chapter introduces the theories underlying government regulation and, in particular, highlights the public interest and public choice approaches.

Learning objectives

By the end of this chapter you should be able to:

- outline the theories of government behaviour and economic regulation
- list the main tools of government intervention
- give examples of the factors which may constrain or promote the regulatory process in health care
- describe the role of interest groups in the regulation process.

Key terms

Capture (self-interest) theory This regards regulation as being supplied in response to the demand of interest groups.

Government failure When the objective of public policy action is undermined by the diverging interests of decision makers within government.

Public choice theory This sees government action as a product of the interaction between voters, politicians and bureaucrats.

Public interest approach In contrast to public choice theory, this approach sees government action as the necessary means of addressing market failures and/or the inability of markets to achieve certain social objectives.

Theories of government behaviour

There are two theories of government behaviour: the public interest approach and public choice theory.

Public interest approach

The *public interest approach* is predicated on the notion that government intervention, particularly regulation, is required to correct for either failures of the market
or the inability of markets to achieve certain social objectives such as equity. A
public interest approach is often used to justify the provision of what are seen to be
merit goods, such as education and health care, by the state.

Public choice theory

Public choice theory takes a different approach. The theory shows that solutions
adopted in response to market failure do not arise from some abstract and monolithic 'public interest' but from the interests of the actors involved and are influenced by the private costs and benefits they confer. As a consequence, the
behaviour of the public sector is viewed as the outcome of interaction between
individual choices made by voters, politicians and bureaucrats. In effect, it tends to
allow for the possibility that these may not be consistent with the achievement of
the government's social objectives, leading to the possibility of *government failure*.
The criticism of this approach is that it tends to assume only self-interest as a
motivating factor. However, individuals working in public sector organizations
are often drawn, and motivated in their work, by broader social and altruistic
concerns. Le Grand (1997) provides a neat discussion of the interaction between
self-interest and social imperatives in public sector decision making.

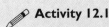

Activity 12.1

The following passage from Jan (2003) examines the problem of translating health
economics research into policy from a public choice perspective. After arguing that
economic analysis by its very nature often creates potential winners and losers in
terms of resources allocation, Jan goes on to suggest possibilities based on agency
theory.

As you read it, consider the following questions:

1 How does the author view the resource allocation problem?
2 What ways are suggested for overcoming this?
3 Can you think of other issues, particularly for low and middle income countries, that
   may also hamper the implementation of policy?

Why does economic analysis not get implemented?

The failure to implement decisions based on economic criteria arises essentially because
within a resource constrained environment, such decisions, in altering the status quo,
inevitably create 'winners' and 'losers'. Indeed, even in instances of expanding budgets,
the allocation of 'new resources' can often lead to the perception that those managers
who have not gained as much as others have instead 'lost' . . . In situations such as these
where decision-making creates 'losers' – actual or perceived – change will invariably be
resisted.

Implementation failure is often attributable to what could be termed simply as the 'failure of will'. This occurs at the level of the decision-maker and relates to a lack of willingness to 'accept . . . responsibility for what may be unpopular choices' . . . and may be exacerbated if the decision-maker needs to maintain close ongoing working relations with those managers and other individuals who will directly 'lose' from an allocation decision. In these circumstances, the explicitness of economic analysis and its emphasis on opportunity costs can compound this problem by identifying more clearly where the losses from decision-making lie . . .

In effect this type of decision-making imposes certain 'decision costs' on the decision-maker . . . Decision costs . . . are associated with a natural aversion to making difficult or uncomfortable decisions . . .

Such costs reflect the inherent conflict of interests, particularly across managers, created by resource allocation decisions of this nature. Within this institutional setting, there is a tendency to resist change and, depending on the decision-making power wielded by potential losers and the decision costs imposed on decision-makers, a degree of inertia in policy making. Furthermore, it can establish a form of 'implementation bias' whereby decisions that are contrary to the interests of groups with greater voice tend, all else being equal, not to be implemented (and vice versa) . . .

Conventional agency theory would suggest that this could be addressed through designing reward systems, along with appropriate monitoring and attribution, that will encourage utility maximizing agents to make decisions that will promote the interests of the principal in response to information asymmetry . . . The aim would be to achieve Pareto-efficient contracts where the agent is remunerated to at least the level that will compensate him/ her for the costs incurred in carrying out the contract and where there are expected residual gains to the principal. In the context of the problem raised in this paper, this raises two possibilities.

Firstly, the decision-makers could be personally remunerated to a level that compensates at least to the level of the decision costs associated with making 'hard decisions'. This measure alone may be effective only if, at the level of the manager, potential losers do not exercise some right of veto. In these instances, implementation would not fail because of the difficulty of extracting 'hard decisions' from decision-makers but from the inherent clash of interests involved in this type of decision and the failure of this measure to address the more fundamental constraint, namely, the resistance from prospective losers.

Instead, a second possibility might be to provide financial incentives directly to managers to accept decisions that might result in cuts to their budgets. This could reduce decision costs thus making easier the job of the decision-maker, but could also compromise the manager's role as an agent for their particular programme area. Such a role is often central to the functioning and cohesion of an organisation since a manager can, not unreasonably, be viewed also as a representative of the interests of his/her particular section, department or programme area in their dealings with higher management. Therefore to offer personal inducements to managers to accept cuts, in effect, creates further conflict of interest through multiple agency. It is conceivable that paying a manager to accept budget cuts and consequently, say, job losses in his/her department is viewed as a 'sell-out' and thus will severely hamper his/her future ability to manage.

The limitations of these measures are that they overlook some of the broader behavioural constraints (e.g. decision costs, multiple agency relations and informal relations) between individuals that tend to extend beyond the scope of conventional agency theory.

Institutional measures that focus on the more general 'rules of the game' as opposed to simply individual financial incentives are therefore the basis for potentially more effective solutions. These entail broad changes to the way the decision-making problem is framed and [are] aimed at both promoting incentive compatibility and building on existing relations and norms of conduct between parties.

As mentioned previously, the problem centres on the one-shot zero sum nature of decision-making. Transforming the institutional setting into one that is more conducive to implementation through incentive measures can be achieved by establishing some form of repetition . . . This represents an application of the well-known Folk Theorem . . . which indicates that the prospects of co-operation are generally increased in repeated games since the likelihood of any one player recouping short-term losses in future is reinforced. The key in this situation is establishing appropriate conditions to enable this type of game to be played out. Such repetition is an important condition for enabling an organization to institute means of sharing the potential efficiency gains (or at least creating the perception of this) across individual departments, programme areas, etc. over the long term. Further-more, even if each separate decision results in a perceived zero sum reallocation, repetition may nonetheless encourage prospective 'losers' to co-operate since an inefficient pro-gramme in one period may subsequently be efficient in another (and vice versa since constant returns to scale within competing programme areas cannot generally be assumed in practice). Thus the identity of a loser in one round will not necessarily be the same in subsequent rounds, thereby creating the prospect of losses sustained in the short term being recouped in the future. This suggests that individual resource allocation decisions are ideally, from the point of view of implementation, linked to ongoing programs of reform rather than viewed as one-off initiatives. Furthermore, the link to future rounds needs to be made explicit so as to minimise the influence of any inherent myopia or bounded rationality of players . . .

In a recent study of decision-making, a consultative process, involving various meetings and procedures for information feedback, was important in promoting co-operation amongst ostensibly competing interests. In these circumstances it was both the informal relations between the managers involved in this process and, importantly, the perceived degree of procedural fairness embodied in decision-making (and not necessarily incentive compati-bility in a strict sense) that was instrumental in determining how well any such co-operative outcome could be sustained amongst players . . . In these circumstances, a degree of goodwill established through a process of consultation was seen as important in offsetting some of the costs of decision-making as well as negotiating the threat of veto held by each of those parties potentially affected by an ensuing decision. The aim of the consultation process, however, was not to induce individuals to abandon self-interest, but to encourage them to be more sophisticated in their pursuit of it by giving them a broader appreciation of the 'political constraints' on decision-making and the potential benefits of co-operation.

In circumstances such as these, co-operation is held together by norms of behaviour that appeal more to a sense of shared values rather than simply mutual self-interest, narrowly defined, but ultimately also have significant economic value in reducing decision costs . . .

Therefore while incentive compatibility is likely to be a significant consideration in terms of how well such co-operation binds . . . the establishment of economic incentives also needs to be done in recognition of the potential effect they may have in altering the culture of decision-making. It is the analysis of these institutional characteristics therefore that allows implementation as a topic to fall within the compass of economic analysis and correspondingly brings in an added perspective to the formulation and evaluation of policy responses to this issue.

 Feedback

> 1 The paper views the resource allocation problem as a process that typically is carried out across a number of programme areas. Each programme has an individual manager in charge of a budget. The assumption is that each manager will tend to resist any proposed cuts to his or her budget. The decision maker's responsibility in this context is to determine the allocation of resources across programmes, thereby creating winners and losers among those managers whose budgets will be altered. Resistance from the potential losers can be seen to impose costs on decision makers and thus provide some explanation for the non-implementation of ostensibly efficiency-enhancing initiatives. This example illustrates the potential tensions between achieving a desired organizational objective and the interests of certain managers.
>
> 2 In deriving solutions, it is useful to view this as a collective action problem (which was discussed in the previous chapter). From the point of view of the organization, implementing economic analysis should lead to greater efficiency and therefore be in the long term interests of managers as a group. A solution would, in effect, require managers to be prepared to accept possible cuts to their budget in the interests of the organization. Achieving this can often require commitment that this process is repeated and ongoing rather than one-off, so that individuals do see the prospects of long term gains offsetting possible short term losses. The paper also recognizes that non-rationalistic norms may also have an impact and that solutions to decision making constraints may involve addressing such norms.
>
> 3 Although not exclusive to low and middle income countries, issues of corruption and a lack of managerial capacity and resources can also be seen to be a major constraint on the implementation of government policies. The author focused mainly on incentive constraints, but in some settings such governance issues can have a major bearing.

Economic theories of regulation

How do the two concepts of government behaviour enable you to understand a specific form of government action, namely, regulation? The two perspectives applied to the analysis of regulation can be labelled the public interest approach and capture or self-interest theory.

The public interest approach

The public interest approach holds that regulation is supplied in response to the demand by the public for the correction of inefficient or inequitable market practices. For instance, the theory tends to promote the regulation of monopolies to restrict prices and ensure adequate supply and quality.

Critics of this approach question the notion of government as a costless and dependably effective instrument for altering market behaviour. A serious problem with the theory is that there is no mechanism to link public interest with legislative action which maximizes public welfare (Posner 1974). That is to say, this theory ignores the inherently political nature of the decision making process.

Capture or self-interest theory

The alternative, *capture* or *self-interest theory*, holds that regulation is influenced by the demands of diverse interest groups. It is based broadly on a public choice perspective of government and was formally developed by Stigler (1971). It suggests that the nature and scope of regulation are the result of the demand by economic and political interests.

The key concept behind this theory is that because influence activities are not costless, regulation tends to favour specialized interest groups as opposed to larger groups representing more diffuse interests because the latter tend to be beset more by collective action (or free-rider) problems.

There have been attempts to test which theory is more appropriate in the context of licensing doctors and other health care professionals. One study (Paul 1984) looked at the decision of American states to license doctors and rejected the public interest theory. It found a strong negative relationship between the year of licensure and the per-capita number of doctors in a state, suggesting that doctors were in a strong position to delay licensing.

Graddy (1991) looked at the regulation of six health care professions (dietician, nurse midwife, occupational therapist, physician assistant, psychologist and social worker). She examined variables related to the public interest (education requirements) and the variables representing the political environment (strength of the majority party) as well as the private interest of the occupations (size of occupation and membership in a professional association). Graddy found that there was a higher probability of a stricter form of regulation in those states where the requirements for professional education were particularly stringent, thus providing support to the public interest motive for regulation.

Propper (1995) raises the issue of regulatory capture, that is, when the regulating agency has close association with the regulated and thus may be more sympathetic towards them. Essentially, this is described as a situation where the regulatee 'captures' or takes control of the regulator and sets the regulatory process to work on their behalf. In the UK, the Department of Health does some regulating but also deals with professional groups in other capacities. For example, the Department has policy targets which may mean that its decisions with regard to furthering competition (e.g. allowing entry) may be compromised – hence the need for an independent regulator. Perhaps the most important policy example in the UK relating to regulatory capture in recent years has been how the Ministry of Agriculture, Fisheries and Food was seen to be 'captured' by powerful industry groups and the National Farmers Union and so failed in its role to deal with the 'mad cow disease' (BSE) crisis.

Activity 12.2

1 What is the key drawback of the public interest approach?
2 Who drives the demand for regulation in the public interest approach and the capture or self-interest theory?
3 What is the key concept behind the capture or self-interest theory?

 Feedback

1 The public interest approach does not take account of the various influences that interest groups have on the decision making process.

2 Public interest theory assumes government action is required by default as a means of addressing the limitations of markets in achieving social goals. The capture or self-interest theory puts emphasis on the role of various interest groups in the design and implementation of regulatory measures.

3 The key concept is that lobbying the regulators is a costly activity and, in contrast to special interest groups, larger groups representing more diffuse interests are less effective as they tend to be beset by collective action problems. It is based on a public choice perspective. However, as discussed earlier, the problem with this approach is that it may overemphasize the role of self-interest, in practice, as a motivating factor within public sector organizations.

The regulatory environment and its constraints

Recent theoretical developments have tried to extend the public choice perspective to reflect the regulatory environment and examine the constraints that prevent the regulator from implementing preferred policies (Laffont and Tirole 1993). Key constraints include:

- *Information.* Does the regulator have sufficient information to determine if there has been a violation? How costly is it to acquire the information? This asymmetry of information may lead to circumstances where the firm tries to extract a rent from its interaction with the government even if its bargaining power is low.
- *Transaction costs.* In the establishment of contracts between parties not all possible contingencies can be covered. This results in uncertainties in the contracting environment which can be seen as transaction costs.
- *Administrative and political constraints.* Regulators may not be free to use any instrument they choose. Regulators themselves may be agents for politicians and follow particular administrative procedures.

It is clear that the process by which regulation is developed and implemented is highly political. If you view regulation as an inherently political process, balancing the competing interests of different actors, it is important to understand the impact of these groups on the design and implementation of regulatory measures.

Regulation and role of interest groups

Although for analytical purposes you have considered economic models of perfect competition, health care markets tend to be imperfect and private and public action have always been interwoven. Evans (1997) argues that redistributional policies have always driven health sector regulation and that 'the notion that some sort of automatic, self-regulating market-like structure can be established that will substitute for public management and yet achieve public objectives' is a fantasy. He examines the debate about competition and regulation and points to the fact that it is difficult to ignore who benefits most from market mechanisms in health care. Taking the example of the USA, he demonstrates the natural alliance between service providers and people with higher incomes. Thus the promotion of market mechanisms needs to be considered in the light that it addresses middle class needs and yields distributional advantages for these influential groups, such as:

- higher incomes for providers
- costs related to use by the wealthier and healthier people
- improved quality without cross-subsidization of the poor.

Evans thus argues that 'distributional questions may be suppressed in economic analysis, but they remain at the forefront of public policy debates'.

 Activity 12.3

Consider the key interest groups and the role that each has to play in your health care system. How might they affect the regulation-setting process?

 Feedback

You will have found that regulation is an inherently political process, balancing the interests of different actors. Actors can include individual patients, consumer groups and organizations, government departments, professional associations, and other agencies that may be involved in the design and implementation of regulatory interventions or who are affected by it.

A key relationship is the one between the regulator (and any intermediaries that are used) and those who are being regulated. For example, professional bodies are often responsible for implementing and enforcing professional standards.

Summary

You have learned about theories of government behaviour: first, the public interest approach that characterizes government as a monolithic and benevolent actor; and second, capture' or 'self-interest' theory where government action (including regulation) is seen as a product of the political process and the interaction of potentially competing interests. You have also seen that regulation cannot be examined in isolation from the political, social and economic context in which it exists. The relative power of interest groups in formulating and shaping regulation, and the interactions of different regulatory mechanisms, once implemented, can be important, as are the intrinsic motivations of decision makers. Understanding the regulatory process in a country requires therefore that the nature of specific institutions, political structures and actors are taken into account.

References

Evans RG (1997) Going for the gold: the redistributive agenda behind market based health care. *Journal of Health Politics, Policy and Law* 22(2): 427–65.

Graddy E (1991) Interest groups or the public interest – why do we regulate health occupations? *Journal of Health Politics, Policy and Law* 16(1): 25–49.

Jan S (2003) Why does economic analysis in health care not get implemented more? Towards a greater understanding of the rules of the game and the costs of decision making. *Applied Health Economics and Health Policy* 2(1): 17–24.

Le Grand J (1997) Knights, knaves or pawns? Human behaviour and social policy. *Journal of Social Policy* 26: 149–69

Laffont J-J and Tirole J (1993) *A Theory of Incentives in Procurement and Regulation*. Cambridge, MA: MIT Press.

Paul C (1984) Physician licensure and the quality of medical care. *Atlantic Economic Journal* 12: 18–30.

Posner RA (1974) Theories of economic regulation. *Bell Journal of Economics and Management Science* 5(2): 335–58.

Propper C (1995) Agency and incentives in the NHS internal market. *Social Science & Medicine* 40: 1683–90.

Stigler GJ (1971) The theory of economic regulation. *Bell Journal of Economics and Management Sciences* 2: 3–21.

SECTION 4

Contracts and agency

Institutional economics and appropriate contracts

Overview

In this chapter you will look at characteristics of transactions, the factors that leave them vulnerable to opportunism, and the governance and contracting approaches that might be used to protect them. Specific examples of contracting are provided and the role of moral hazard and adverse selection is highlighted. Some examples of extending market relationships into health care systems are given.

Learning objectives

After working through this chapter you should be able to:

- explain the theories relating to the existence of firms
- understand transaction costs
- identify situations in which 'opportunistic' behaviour might arise
- explain how moral hazard and adverse selection affect the appropriate form of contracting
- identify appropriate measures to improve contracts for the health sector
- describe some of the evidence relating to contracts in reformed health sectors.

Key terms

Governance The means by which order is accomplished in a relation in which potential conflict threatens to undo or upset opportunities to realize mutual gains.

What is institutional economics?

The aim of institutional economics (or, more precisely, a strand known as new institutional economics which is the focus of this chapter), like that of neoclassical economics, is the efficient use of resources: it is concerned with maximization and the costs of conducting a transaction. The task in institutional economics is not merely to minimize production costs but to minimize both production costs and transaction costs. This minimization, in many circumstances, will require governance structures that differ from the governance by markets assumed in neoclassical economics. Governance may be enforced in hierarchies or organized in networks or in some hybrid form of arrangement. Institutional economics provides a framework in which to assess the appropriateness of different forms of governance.

The concept of transaction costs is at the heart of the new institutional economics developed in the work of Oliver Williamson. He defined transaction costs as concerned with 'an examination of the comparative costs of planning, adapting and monitoring task completion under alternative governance structures'.

Transaction costs can be incurred ex ante or ex post. Ex-ante costs occur before the contract is implemented. These involve the costs of drafting, negotiating and safeguarding the contract. Ex-post transaction costs occur once the execution of the contract is in place. An ex-post cost may consist of monitoring the work, resolution of disputes and renegotiating contracts when necessary.

The concept of transaction costs is attributed to Commons (1931) and Coase (1937) who sought to explain the existence of firms. The existence of firms was considered to be a response not only to technological features such as economies of scale and scope, but also to the relative costs of producing internally compared with the cost of buying in goods from others. This cost of buying in would include the cost of setting up the transaction and ensuring its completion. The boundary of an organization or firm is defined as the line across which only price-mediated transactions take place. Inside the boundary, firms make decisions in a managerial or hierarchical manner.

Whether transactions are organized within a firm hierarchically or between autonomous firms in the market depends upon the nature of the transaction costs associated with that transaction:

> A transaction cost occurs when a good or service is transferred across a technologically separable interface. One stage of activity terminates and another begins. With a well-working interface, as with a well-working machine, these transfers occur smoothly. (Williamson 1985)

The definition of transaction costs provided by Cotter (1989) is perhaps somewhat clearer:

> Broadly conceived, transaction costs refer to any use of resources required to negotiate and enforce agreements, including the costs of information needed to formulate a bargaining strategy, the time spent haggling, and the costs of preventing cheating by the parties to the bargain.

As Buckley and Chapman (1997) point out, transaction costs can also be viewed as the costs that would have been incurred had the transaction not been properly set up:

> Transaction costs are funny things: the most important of them exist not in reality but in the realities that have been avoided in worlds that have not come to be.

Activity 13.1

What form of transaction costs would you envisage being associated with setting up contracts for the purchase of:

- hospital linen
- X-ray machines
- care for the elderly
- a vaccination programme for children
- ward cleaning?

Distinguish between ex-ante and ex-post transaction costs.

 Feedback

Transaction costs relating to linen and X-ray machines would be associated with specification of the technical requirements and quality controls that should be built into the contract. They would largely be ex ante. Contracts for care of the elderly would require substantial ex-ante and ex-post costs as the contracts could not be completely specified and there would be scope for opportunism in delivery unless the contract was monitored. It should be possible to draw up a fairly comprehensive contract for cleaning but the execution of the contract would need to be monitored as the work might be scrimped or insufficient, or inappropriate cleaning materials may be used.

Opportunism in health care contracts

The major features described in transaction cost economics can be seen in the health sector. The rationality is no doubt bounded as the information requirements are vast and the ability to process and analyse such complex information is likely to be beyond the capacity of those involved. There is, in addition, uncertainty both of the traditional type and the behaviour kind described by Williamson (1985). Asset specificity of all types occurs. So contracting in the health sector is likely to be subject to opportunism.

Adverse selection

One form of ex-ante opportunism is adverse selection. In the context of contracting it may be possible for either party to frame the contract in such a way that the other party bears the risks. The provider may find they have taken on risks associated with patient groups that they thought the purchaser had covered in some other way, while the purchasers may find that the provider has inserted clauses that exclude high cost cases.

Many cases in the contracts and service agreements used in the NHS in the UK are designed to pass on the risks to the providers. Few contingency funds are retained by purchasers against unexpected events, although sometimes providers group together to share risks. By passing on the risk to the providers in this way the purchasers may find that providers select patients they are likely to find easy to treat.

The contracting process is set in the context of other goals that might also give rise to moral hazard. The one that besets the UK health system is the waiting time or waiting list target. To meet the target of waiting times a number of ruses could be used. Patients may not be placed on the list until it is clear that they can be dealt with within the time limit, or they may even be taken off lists if targets seem to be in jeopardy.

Moral hazard

As you learned in Chapter 11, moral hazard refers to behaviour by one party that is prejudicial to the interests of the other and that is facilitated by lack of information or ability to scrutinize the implementation of the contract. The moral hazard in contracts in the reformed health sector often takes the form of cutting corners – doing less than one would expect given the terms of the agreement. This may be true in the case of cleaning work done under contract. The problem is accentuated by the nature of the agency relationship that exists between workers and managers. You will learn more about this in the next chapter on agency.

Failure to carry out the terms of a contract means that many health sector activities operate outside a framework of quality assurance and safety controls, all of which increase the transaction costs associated with the governance of the contract.

One of the major problems of contracting in complex situations is that the information needed in the drawing up and scrutinizing of contracts needs to involve those with knowledge of the product who would be able to point to areas where opportunistic behaviour might occur. However, research into the working of managed markets in the area of infectious disease showed that people with the necessary specialist knowledge were not involved, although some were of necessity drawn into ex-post negotiations when there were problems (Allen *et al.* 2002).

The sharing of accretions and depreciation of capital assets should also be determined in the contract, or the parties to a contract may be in jeopardy of being excluded from gains or possible losses that should have been shared. In the early phase of privatization, contracts transferring assets largely failed to add clauses about the distribution of gains and losses in the short term. As a result some entrepreneurial purchasers stood to gain large amounts as the true market value of their purchases became known.

Allen *et al.* found that the contractual relationships in the reformed NHS could only be understood in the context of the organizational arrangements, practices of what they perceived to be the 'continuing relationships in a hierarchy, upon which an internal market structure had been imposed'.

Some of the obvious early failures of contracts have been remedied in later contracting rounds. It takes time to develop a contracting culture in an organization. An understanding of the nature of the product that is being bought or sold should inform contracts. The impact of possible opportunistic behaviour on patients' health should be assessed at each stage of the process.

> Contracting is not cheap. Negotiating, managing and monitoring contracts is expensive: there are high transaction costs. The financial transaction costs are not the only ones. There are clinical transaction costs associated with delays and distortions to patients' care. These arise because of problems of defining responsibility and determining the boundaries of contracts. Unfortunately, any

hope that clinical care could take place uninterrupted in situations in which prices and contracts have to be arranged was misplaced. Purchasers are in the invidious situation of having to agree priorities and ration care to individuals. (Roberts 1993)

The effect of opportunistic behaviour on equity also needs to be monitored. It should be acknowledged that there are difficulties in contracting that call for a different form of governance.

Checking contracts

It is important to scrutinize contracts for possible ways in which opportunism might affect the parties to the contract and those needing health care. Some questions that might be posed when looking at contracts are as follows:

- Will the care contracted for be comprehensive?
- Will it be efficiently delivered?
- Are there any incentives to avoid high cost groups?
- Are there opportunities to cut corners and undertreat?
- Will the arrangements delay patient care?
- Are the parts of the contract that need to be complete well specified?
- Are the contracts capable of modification if unforeseen circumstances arise?
- Will the contracts stifle or stimulate innovation?

 Activity 13.2

1 How might you explore whether adverse selection was taking place in your local hospital?
2 How might you monitor the performance of a cleaning contract for your hospital that has been troubled by outbreaks of hospital-acquired infection?

 Feedback

1 It might show itself in the case mix. It may be that the hospital creams off the simple cases with few co-morbidities, leaving the more complex cases to wait longer or be sent elsewhere.

2 It is important that some governance structure is adopted that can build up an agency relationship with the cleaners to ensure that good practice is implemented. In the UK the failure of the early contracting system for cleaning hospitals has been recognized by the appointment of 'modern matrons' who have responsibility and authority to see that good practice cleaning takes place.

Contracts and efficiency gains

One of the central issues that must be faced when evaluating reformed health systems revolves around whether or not contracting will improve efficiency: will technological and transaction costs be minimized?

Transaction cost economics suggests that the form of organization should be such that costs are minimized. The choice between internal organization via governance within the firm and contracts between firms mediated by the price system should, under this framework, depend upon the characteristics of the transaction and the relationships between the parties. If it appears that in some circumstances, in spite of the most careful contracting and monitoring systems, the organization would still be subject to unacceptable amounts of risk or opportunism and thus face very high transaction costs, then internal organization within a vertically integrated firm may be the most appropriate form of organization. The contractual system becomes too complex.

But to what extent do serious difficulties with the contracting exist within a health care system? The structures of health care organizations are rarely determined by the underlying economic factors, either technological or transactional. To some extent the structures are determined by decree. This has certainly been the case in the UK which, until recently, could be seen as a mostly vertically integrated system. The scheme for quasi-markets was structured to a large extent by decree. The purchaser and provider split was a structure imposed, not determined, by the evidence relating to the minimization of transaction and production costs. Few studies have been carried out to estimate the savings to be made from provider competition. Even if it were possible to find gains from the contracting processes, it is unclear who is benefiting from such gains and who is losing.

The accountability of agents in the system of provider markets is often very weak, with little attention being paid to motivation or property rights. You will explore these issues in Chapter 15 on agency.

 Activity 13.3

Under what conditions is contracting more likely to be effective than public sector provision?

 Feedback

Public services often fail to assess the potential for improving the service internally before resorting to contracting out. Few contracting parties in the public sector have the skills needed to design and monitor contracts. In many countries the basic legal and banking infrastructure is not robust enough to guard against corruption and patronage.

Summary

You have looked at the application of concepts from institutional economics to the issues that surround health sector activity and policy. The weaknesses in contracting have been discussed. Many of these can be remedied by better informed and skilled contractors, but some are embedded in the nature of the transaction and are not so easy to remedy.

References

Allen PA, Croxson B, Roberts JA, Archibald K, Crawshaw S and Taylor L (2002) The use of contracts in the management of infectious disease related risk in the NHS internal market. *Health Policy* 59: 257–81.

Buckley PJ and Chapman M (1997) The perception and measurement of transaction costs. *Cambridge Journal of Economics* 21.

Coase, R (1937) The nature of the firm. *Economica* 4(13–16): 386–405.

Commons, JR (1931) Institutional economics. *American Economic Review* 21: 648–57.

Cotter (1989) Transaction costs, in Eatwell J, Milgate M and Newman P (eds) *The New Palgrave: Allocation Information and Markets*. Basingstoke: Macmillan.

Roberts JA (1993) Managing markets. *Journal of Public Health Medicine* 15(4): 305–10.

Williamson OE (1985) *The Economic Institutions of Capitalism*. New York: Free Press.

Williamson OE (1996) *The Mechanisms of Governance*. New York: Oxford University Press.

14 Legal and economic analysis of contracts

Overview

In the previous chapter you examined the conceptual foundations for the economic analysis of contracts. In this chapter you will consider more specifically some of their legal and economic aspects. The issues discussed are the characteristics of legally binding contracts, freedom of contract, allocation of risk and the characteristics of relational contracts. You will also use some of the ideas from institutional economics to help you consider circumstances that influence governance structures and thus the usefulness of the contracting process.

Learning objectives

At the end of the chapter you should be able to:

- **explain the concept of contract from legal and economic perspectives**
- **explain the difference between neoclassical and institutional economics in the context of contract.**

Key terms

Asset specificity Characteristics of assets that determine whether they are redeployable or not. There are four types of asset specificity: site, physical asset, human asset, and dedicated asset.

Bliss A transaction in which parties engage to their mutual advantage using a classical contract.

Bounded rationality Behaviour that is intendedly rational, but only limitedly so. There are limits of knowledge and capacity that compromise efforts to behave rationally.

Opportunism Situation where one party involved in a contract acts in his or her self-interest at the expense of the other party.

Uncertainty Situation in which it is not possible to know or even predict the likelihood of an event occurring. This notion is distinguished from that of 'risk', where probabilities are known.

The contract: a legal perspective

How contract law is encoded in your country will depend on the prevailing civil law tradition. In countries with an Anglo-Saxon tradition, such as the UK and USA, civil law is based on common law that is mainly contained in precedents set by cases decided in the courts over the past several hundred years, as amended by statutes (Furmston 1996). In countries with a Roman law tradition, such as most other European countries and countries in the French- and Spanish-speaking world, contract law is laid down in the civil code. It is not necessary to go into detail about the law of contract, but you will look at some of the universal principles that apply to contracts in general to enable you to understand some of their economic implications.

You could take this discussion as an opportunity to find out more about the legal principles that apply in your own country.

Characteristics of a legally binding contract

Certain preconditions have to apply before an agreement can have the status of a legally binding contract. These include:

- a clear offer and acceptance (so that a meeting of minds can be said to have occurred)
- the absence of coercion
- the intention to create legal relations (unlike promises made in domestic circumstances, for example)
- the giving of 'consideration' in return for the promise to perform (i.e. the act or promise offered by one party and accepted by the other as the price of that other's promise).

Freedom of contract

The important point to note from an economic point of view is that the basic tenet is *freedom of contract*. This means that parties can make any bargain they like, and the courts will not enquire into whether it was a good bargain (the courts are not concerned with the adequacy of consideration).

This is linked to the idea that a free market in which choice is exercised by consumers in accordance with their individual utility functions will be allocatively efficient. This idea is often expressed using the analogy, as discussed in earlier chapters, of the 'invisible hand' that in a free market ensures the optimum allocation of goods and services. Parties must be free not to make a contract at all if they do not wish to: they should not be coerced. A contract will not be legally binding if each party has not entered into it of their own free will.

Allocation of risk

The point of making a legally binding contract is to allocate risk in advance. Both parties agree as to how risk will be borne in the future. This occurs because the terms of the original contract (which may or may not be written) will be used as the primary set of rules to decide who should bear the risk in the circumstances then pertaining. Were a dispute to arise, the court would look at the original terms to decide who should bear the risk, not at what might be fair in the present situation.

Over and above that, the law of contract itself consists of rules which are also known in advance. Because a contract is legally binding a party can invoke the machinery of the state, via the courts, to enforce its terms.

In drawing up a contract that will enable you to allocate risk and then enforce your rights effectively, it is necessary to cover the following areas adequately:

- specification of performance (quantity, and quality if this is a concern)
- how products or services will be priced
- how performance will be monitored.

You can see from this description that the classical law of contract works on the principle that it is possible to be certain about all future events, so that they can all be catered for in the agreement. The agreement must be complete.

Relational contracts

In many circumstances the description of the contract contained in classical law, as set out above, is adequate. Such contracts tend to be for simple transactions where performance is easily ascertained, such as the purchase of a batch of syringes or a tin of beans from the corner shop, or for situations that can be specified in great detail and easily monitored. They are discrete: 'sharp in by clear agreement, sharp out by clear performance' (Macneil 1978). There are circumstances, however, in which it is not possible to draw up a 'complete contract'. There may be uncertainty about the expected level of activity or costs over the contracting period, or there may be measurement problems associated with assessing perform-ance. In such situations parties agree to 'open up' contracts if unexpected events or problems occur; specific or general clauses may qualify the terms of the contract. These contracts will then be dependent on relationships between the parties and the trust they invest in each other. They are often referred to as relational contracts.

Compared to classical contracts, relational contracts are:

- not discrete – the commencement and termination may not be determined in the written contract
- not complete – not all elements can be specified and measured
- likely to be adjusted or varied
- dependent on personal relationships, trust and cooperation.

The legal definition of a complete contract fits in well with the concept of a transaction in the marketplace envisaged by neoclassical economics. In contrast to the way in which contracts had conventionally been conceptualized by legal and economic scholars, 'some contract law specialists and some economists were becoming more interested in phenomena in which continuity between unchanging parties to a contract was a source of productive value' (Williamson 1996).

Contracts and markets

Parties to contracts in competitive and contestable markets can rely upon market disciplines to ensure that contracts are efficiently priced. Although contracts, being at the heart of exchange theory, are very important for economic analysis, they are not explored fully in neoclassical economic theory. This theory fails to explore the 'black box' of the contract or agreement made between those who buy and those who sell. Traditional economics assumes bargains will be struck between buyers and sellers using signals which emanate from the price system without imposing costs: they emerge from a 'frictionless system' of trading.

What causes problems in contracting?

In a perfectly competitive market where information is complete, there is certainty that trade can take place in a perfectly frictionless way. Parties can, by offering to buy or sell a good or service in exchange for something of value, contract to their mutual advantage. They are also free to walk away if the terms of the transaction are not acceptable. It is quite appropriate to use a classical contract having the properties outlined earlier. This is the situation that Williamson has dubbed *bliss*.

In other situations Williamson recognizes that there may be contractual difficulties. In situations in which bounded rationality, uncertainty or asset specificity exist it will not be easy to achieve a mutually satisfactory contract or to walk away. In case of asset specificity, for example, the value of the asset in any alternative use will be low, thus exposing the provider to losses if the contract does not go ahead. Alternatively, the special nature of the asset might leave the consumer without an alternative source of supply if the contract is not implemented. The ability of either party to walk away will be severely limited. Where there is lack of information and uncertainty it is possible for even high minded honest organizations to be invaded and exploited by unscrupulous agents. In situations such as these, trust and relationships are valued. Adjustments to meet certain contingencies or more general adjustments may be a feature of the contracting process.

If neither general nor specific clause contracts are likely to ensure the transaction, then the organization may decide that the most satisfactory and efficient strategy would be to integrate (usually vertically) with another organization or to expand the existing organization. In such situations the governance structure of the organization will change from a *market* to a *hierarchy*.

Identifying conditions in which contracts may be vulnerable to 'opportunistic' behaviour

Williamson delineates the ease or difficulty in maintaining market relations using a matrix to illustrate the effect of lack of information and the presence of opportunism (Table 14.1). Let us explore each of these situations.

Table 14.1 Different contractual environments

		Condition of bounded rationality	
		Absent	*Admitted*
Condition of opportunism	*Absent*	Bliss	'General clause' contracting
	Admitted	Comprehensive contracting	Contractual difficulties

Source: Williamson (1985)

Bliss

Where there is unbounded rationality and no possibility of opportunistic behaviour (largely because it occurs in a perfect market where parties are free to walk away and sellers are price takers, not price makers) then the normal classical contract will suffice.

 Activity 14.1

Think of some examples where such 'blissful' contracts might be suitable for purchasing health care.

 Feedback

The health facility would be able to enter into 'blissful' contracts for general items such as stationery, office equipment, hospital beds and electricity supply. The health facility will have knowledge of such items (so there is no bounded rationality) and be able to judge whether the contract has been fulfilled. Parties to the contract will not be subject to great uncertainties, the contracts will tend to be repeated and thus the tendency for opportunism will be minimized.

Comprehensive contracting

Unbounded rationality or perfect information informs a contract of this type. It can be safeguarded by specifying in great detail all that is expected from the parties to it. Its implementation can be monitored to ensure that it has been carried out as agreed. This is another example where complete classical contracts would be suitable.

 Activity 14.2

Give some examples of purchasing health care for which a comprehensive contract might be drawn up.

Feedback

> Any contract for which it is possible to specify the exact requirements and monitor whether these have been met would meet the requirements of a comprehensive contract. The health facility might order some X-ray machines, for example, the detailed specifications for which can be laid out clearly and monitored by technical staff.

General clause contracting

This form of contract will work in situations where, although there is incomplete information, there is no opportunism. This works well because the general clauses protect against incompleteness of contracting events that could not be predicted.

This might be an appropriate way to contract for doctors' services, where precise specifications may not be possible in advance. Often general clause contracts are modified or constrained by setting limits on quantity or cost beyond which renegotiation becomes necessary. An example of such a clause was found in a contract for medical services in Scotland which had throughput targets. These were compromised following a large infectious disease outbreak that used up all available renal beds for children for many weeks, thus reducing the throughput of other cases. However, a clause had been inserted requesting that the purchasers should be informed of any unexpected events. This was done and so the funds were made available. In the same outbreak, however, providers with no such clause in their contracts, mainly providers of laboratory services, had to absorb the extra costs although at the time of the outbreak it was proclaimed that all that could be done should be done. Such failure to recognize the expense and effort involved in dealing with the extra workload could have jeopardized trust and fractured future relationships between the health care purchasers and the pathology departments (Roberts *et al.* 2000).

Serious contractual difficulties

These occur when there is bounded rationality, opportunism and incomplete information.

Types of contract

Those seeking appropriate contracts need to be aware of the distribution of risks that arise in different forms of contract. There are three basic models of contract: block contracts, cost and volume contracts, and cost-per-case contracts. You will look at these contracts in the light of the framework that has been developed using new institutional economics.

Block contracts

Funds are transferred in much the same way as a budget, and the provider is given the responsibility for carrying out all the work that arises within the description of the contract. In this sense it has characteristics of a general clause contract, but it is often limited in the same way as a cash-limited budget. The financial risks fall on the provider which may find it does not have sufficient funds to carry out all the work. This may result from the uncertainty in the prediction of the demand for services or from a shift in the case mix. A provider intent upon keeping within its budget may ration care as far as possible within the terms of the agreement. Ultimately the risk is borne by the patients who may not get treated or who have to wait. Such rationing may be unfair. Those presenting early in the contracting period may have a better chance of being seen, unless proper management procedures are in place to ration funds appropriately throughout the period of the contract. The provider may hide behind the block contract and do as little as possible, perhaps switching activity to cases that yield more revenue. There may be a moral hazard problem.

Cost and volume contracts

These contracts can counteract some of the problems associated with budgets (as in block contracts). A block of money may be transferred as before, but the volume expected is now specified. These contracts may contain clauses that trigger extra payments in certain situations. Such arrangements are a version of the two-tier pricing policy that has traditionally been used to ensure that large fixed costs are covered, for instance in the electricity industry. In this case the risks are reduced for the provider and the patient, but the financial implications for the purchaser are more difficult to predict.

Cost-per-case contracts

A cost-per-case (or fee-for-service (FFS)) contract is one in which the provider undertakes to treat each patient for a fee (agreed prospectively or retrospectively). Retrospective billing exposes health systems to cost escalation and leads to pressure for prospective fee structures – for example, using the diagnostic related group system of charging in USA and reference price charging in the UK. It is not possible, however, to fix both price and quantity, and providers facing a fixed fee per case may seek to treat more cases to maintain their income (supplier-induced demand). Fee-for-service (FFS) contracts tend to expose purchasers to budgetary pressure, but by attaching funding to individual patients in this way, adequate care for underprivileged groups could be ensured.

 Activity 14.3

A purchaser has decided to pay on a cost-per-case basis for treating patients in primary care. What advice would you give them on the issues that might arise for treating chronic illness, vaccination and an acute case of asthma?

 Feedback

You should consider whether the self-interest of the provider would lead to more appointments with the chronically sick or not. If so, what would the likely benefits be to the patient and to the provider? Monitoring may reduce incidents of acute illness and maintain the patient better. A cost-per-case basis for vaccination may increase the vaccination take-up rate, but the provider may find it took more effort to attract those most at risk and so the preventive effect may be modified. Paying for treatment of a case of acute asthma would possibly improve care if the nearest hospital was some distance away, but would possibly require more technology and training and provide less effective care.

Summary

You have learned the concept of a legally binding contract, the factors necessary to establish a legally binding contract and the importance of allocating risk. Just as there may be problems in establishing a classical contract in the presence of uncertainty, there may also be problems in using the market form of governance for such transactions.

You have also learned about the characteristics – bounded rationality, uncertainty, asset specificity – that have implications for the type of contract used; in particular, they may facilitate opportunistic behaviour. Williamson's matrix was reproduced to illustrate some combinations of bounded rationality and opportunism that have implications for contracting. The typology of contracts and the way in which the different types of contract apportion risk among the parties were illustrated.

References

Furmston M (1996) Cheshire, Fifoot and Furmston's Law of Contract. London: Butterworth.
Macneil IR (1978) Contracts: adjustments of long-term economic relations under classical, neo-classical and relational contract law. Northwestern University Law Review 72(6): 854–905.
Roberts JA, Upton PA and Azene G (2000) Escherichia coli O157:H7; an economic assessment of an outbreak. Journal of Public Health Medicine 22(1): 99–107.
Williamson OE (1985) The Economic Institutions of Capitalism. New York: Free Press.
Williamson OE (1996) The Mechanisms of Governance. New York: Oxford University Press.

Agency and organizational decision making

Overview

Agency relationships impact on the way in which health care is delivered. Much of the focus in this book thus far has been on agency in the context of the doctor–patient relationship, particularly the issues of moral hazard and adverse selection that can arise in this relationship (see Chapters 4 and 11). This topic was also touched upon in Chapter 13 on contracting, where you used the lens of institutional economics to consider the behaviour of the participants and suggested solutions to some of the agency problems that arise. This chapter introduces the concept of agency in greater depth, focusing on the role that agency relationships play in the governance of health care in many reformed health care systems, especially those that adopt an internal market structure or those that employ a mixture of public and private finance and production.

Learning objectives

At the end of this chapter you should be able to:

- **recognize the tensions and conflicts of interest that arise between agents and principals**
- **describe why these tensions or conflicts of interest arise**
- **discuss the implications of trust and altruism for agency relationships.**

Key terms

Agent A person who acts on behalf of another (the principal).

Impacted information When information resides with the agent it may be impacted; there would be high costs to achieving information parity.

Informational asymmetry A principal recognizes his or her own information deficit and the superiority of the agent's information.

Principal A person on whose behalf an agent acts.

The agency relationship

The problems of agency are all-pervasive and not confined to public sector activities. Indeed, as suggested by Arrow (1985), agency represents a significant component of almost all transactions. According to Stiglitz (1990): 'If there are actions which one of the individuals can undertake between the date of the contract and the event that will affect the outcome, then there is a principal–agent relationship between the two.'

The principal–agent concept has been used to explore relationships between managers, who have no share in the property of a company, and shareholders; and to explore the whole hierarchy of relationships within bureaucracies and firms. You will find these problems in all organizational settings where one individual (or firm) hires another to do a specific job. This agency relationship differs from the relationship between buyers and sellers assumed in neoclassical theory, which emphasizes the symmetry in economic relationships (Stiglitz 1990).

The following excerpt from Strong and Waterson (1987) describes agency relationships.

Principals, agents and information

The principal–agent problem characterizes a number of situations where self-interested individuals enter into an implicit or explicit contractual arrangement. Examples of agency relationships are pervasive. An obvious example is between employer and employee, but they extend to other relationships such as those between regulator and regulated, lender and borrower, client and adviser, insurer and insured, and government and governed (although here it is not clear who is principal and who is agent).

The simplest agency model assumes that the principal delegates to the agent the responsibility for selecting and implementing an action. The agent is compensated by the principal, with the principal being the residual claimant to the outcome of the agent's act, after payment of the compensation. The principal's problem is to negotiate a contract specifying the agent's remuneration, knowing that their interests are not in complete harmony. For example, the employer may design a form of wage contract which induces the employee to work hard.

In solving the problem, both principal and agent are assumed to be motivated by self-interest. This means that the agent selects an action given his/her own information and the remuneration scheme, in order to maximize utility. Similarly, the principal selects a remuneration scheme to maximize utility in the light of the agent's self-interested behaviour.

In game-theoretic terms, the principal–agent problem is a two-person non-cooperative (and non-constant sum) game. It is clearly non-constant sum since different actions can give rise to a different total outcome. The non-cooperative description arises from the assumption that principal and agent are driven by self-interest rather than communal interest. Some people . . . see the modern firm as a coalition of interests and therefore discuss relationships between the parties in terms of a *cooperative* bargaining game. This seemingly contrasts with the contractual viewpoint, though the idea that the firm encompasses a collection of interests is common to both. We would argue that it is not clear that the participants in these relationships see themselves as a community of interests.

Activity 15.1

1 What can the study of the agency relationship in terms of firms and organizations help you to understand?
2 What is the key characteristic of both *agent* and *principal* in agency theory?

 Feedback

1 The study of the agency relationship can help you to understand:

- the internal organization of the firm
- the relationship between top decision makers in the firm and the firm's residual owners
- the relationships between the firm and external parties.

2 The key assumed characteristic of both agent and principal is that of self-interested behaviour. Agency is a concept that can be applied to many organizational settings; it is closely related to the theory of the firm. The firm can be thought of as an institution which acquires resources and organizes them to produce an output. Agency is an approach of institutional economics that explicitly considers the behaviour of the participants and suggests solutions to some of the problems that arise from their behaviour.

 Activity 15.2

Give examples of agency from organizational settings you are familiar with and describe the key characteristics of these relationships.

 Feedback

You may have suggested examples such as the relationship between owner and manager, managers and employees, insurer and insured, regulator and regulated, doctor and patient, lawyer and client, and between parties to a contract. In all these relationships the partners have different interests and try to find ways to maximize their utility. All principals expect a specific service to be performed by the agents, which they cannot or do not want to perform themselves. All relationships involve differences in power and information resources.

Agency and management

Managers can be considered to occupy a dual position. They can be seen as agents in relation to some principal (e.g. government or shareholders) or as occupying the role of principals in relation to employees.

It has been suggested that managers in organizations may be increasingly exposed to the agency problem because of:

- the increasing complexity of the environment
- the limited ability of managers
- constraints on the ability of top managers to assimilate information.

In such circumstances, benefits may be obtained by delegating decisions to agents.

The central problem of agency arises because the principal and the agent have:

- different utility functions
- different information sets.

It is expected that the agent will select actions that minimize the impact on their own utility function at the expense of the principal. This is possible because the principal does not have access to all the information available to the agent. So most of the major problems arising from the agency relationship are due to information asymmetry. If the principal and the agent had exactly the same information, moral hazard and adverse selection would not arise.

A problem arises because the principal (owner of the firm) cannot be sure that the agent has used all the information available in performing their role for two reasons:

- the agent's effort cannot be observed
- external factors affect the agent.

This means that because the information is *impacted* (condensed, available to the agent only), the principal has no way of knowing whether it has been properly used. It is then argued that even if the agent's action and the outcome are jointly observed, the principal cannot know whether the action was optimal given the agent's private information.

For example, an employer may not share a worker's information that a higher productivity outcome might have been attained with increased effort, in which case the worker has a strong incentive to suppress the information and economize on effort. On the other hand, the principal must introduce incentives to the agency that ensure that this form of moral hazard is minimized.

 Activity 15.3

What are the possible consequences of moral hazard and adverse selection?

 Feedback

Strong and Waterson (1987) see moral hazard arising 'when the principal and agent share the same information up to the point at which the agent selects an action, but thereafter the principal is only able to observe the outcome or pay-off, not the action itself'. The moral hazard may involve underperformance that cannot be directly observed and may be attributed to 'external factors'.

The simplest form of adverse selection arises when the principal is not privy to some information which is relevant to the action, whereas the agent can make use of this information when selecting an action. The agent knows the action chosen, but the principal is unable to tell from observing the outcome alone which combination of action and state of the world has occurred. Because of this, information about effort is of value to the principal as long as the cost of providing it does not exceed the possible benefits to be gained from its use in the negotiating process.

Activity 15.4

It is a common experience that agents and principals have different utility and information. Assume you are responsible for managing a vaccination programme that is carried out by health workers. What incentives could ensure mitigation of the type of moral hazard discussed above?

Feedback

The principal's task is to design a reward system that will motivate the agent to perform the agency task as well as possible. Given that effort cannot be observed, the principal may have to rely on rewarding according to output. This is sometimes difficult to measure, and measures can be manipulated. If the measure is expressed in items of service, more will be done; if it is expressed in terms of complexity, there will be more complexity. For example, in a salaried scheme with health workers receiving a fixed payment, failure to achieve vaccination targets would not be penalized. The above model would predict that as the actual effort put into achieving the target cannot be observed, the manager (principal) cannot assess the true effort put into the campaign and the agents may blame external factors such as low turnout or lack of supplies for the failure. Under a fee-for-service (FFS) scheme (e.g. the remuneration depending on numbers of children vaccinated) an incentive for increased effort would be introduced. But external factors could still play a role if targets were not achieved.

External factors

The ability to perform an agency depends not only upon the agent's effort but also upon external factors. The environment in which the health sector operates may not be conducive to high performance. The population may be poor, housing may be unsatisfactory, water and sanitation may be far from ideal, and the education level of the population may not be conducive to encouraging cooperative effort or partnership in health care. While all these issues may indeed affect performance, they can also be used to excuse poor results and it may be very difficult to attribute blame or reward success. Those reacting against the imposition of performance indicators almost always explain their relative failure by recourse to external factors (Roberts *et al.* 1998).

The incentive package

In addition to external factors, the compensation package must allow for the agent's attitude to risk taking. Agents who are more risk-averse than principals may need to be compensated for risk taking. The design of an incentive package to motivate agents is part of mechanism design theory. Whatever package is produced, however, there are forces other than the principal that impinge on the behaviour of the agent. These may be internal to the institution concerned, such as the relative performance of other agents, the security of the job or the reputation among peers. Alternatively, they may be external to the institution: labour market conditions or the degree of competition for the services of the agent.

> The principal will not usually be able to scrutinize the work being carried out or determine the factors that contribute to its success or failure. There are risks involved in any undertaking, and the agents will not always be at fault if health care is ineffective. Systems of controls are needed to ensure as far as possible that organizations bear the responsibility for their failings and do not bear the responsibility for factors outside their control. The design of systems to discriminate in this way is extremely difficult, and excuses for poor performance abound. The debate in the United Kingdom about the use of examination results as indicators of performance in education illustrates this problem particularly well. The negotiation of optimal incentive structures, of course, begs the question of whether self-interest does or should propel health care systems. (Roberts 1993)

Motivations other than self-interest are seen as key to the agency relationship, and in health care in particular self-interest is expected to be replaced to some extent by the internalized values of professional ethics which ensure that the agent works in the patients' best interests.

Activity 15.5

Considering public choice agency theory, what other factors or disciplines would you expect to counteract the self-interested behaviour of agents?

Feedback

Public choice agency theory considers that the *market mechanism* will remove informational asymmetries and contain the discretionary power of agents. Some case studies of early endeavours in quasi-markets seem to suggest that market disciplines do work in some areas: cleaning, rubbish collection and so on. But in other areas it is considered by some that the disciplines imposed, such as specific contracts and monitoring of contractual obligations, can be counterproductive and even alienating. It has also been suggested that individuals display loyalty, share value sets and care what others think about their work effort. You could add that they also get enjoyment from their work.

In organizations *group phenomena and conventions* play a large part in shaping individuals' work behaviour. Departures from group norms often lead to informal sanctions. The disciplines are horizontal and delivered by the group. The sanctions prevent free-riding, reduce the scope for moral hazard and limit the scope for discretion and so maintain conventions. But these mechanisms are sometimes modified by internal power relations that preclude some agents from responding to peer pressure even if that pressure is exerted.

Trust

Trust is an important factor of the principal–agent relationship. Where it exists it is seen to enhance efficiency, but it takes time to establish and cannot be substituted for or traded. Trust is very fragile; once lost, it cannot easily be regained. Vertical controls imposed hierarchically, such as sanctions, performance indicators, penalties and incentives, are seen to dilute trust or signal distrust and may increase costs as they are expensive to impose and monitor.

As mentioned above, self-interested behaviour will not necessarily be the only motive of professionals who by the ethics of their profession are expected to be collectively oriented and willing to forgo personal gain for the greater good.

Summary

You have learned about the nature of the principal–agent relationship and how it manifests itself within the firm. In the next chapter you will look more specifically at the nature of agency in terms of health service purchasing and provision, and look again at both economic and non-economic incentives used to address the problem of the principal–agent relationship.

References

Arrow KJ (1985) The economics of agency, in Pratt JW and Zeekhauser RJ (eds) *Principals and Agents: The Structure of Business*, pp. 37–51. Boston, MA: Harvard Business School Press.
Roberts JA (1993) Managing markets. *Journal of Public Health Medicine* 15(4): 305–10.
Roberts JA, Le Grand J and Bartlett W (1998) Lessons from quasi-markets in the 1990s, in Bartlett W, Roberts JA and Le Grand J (eds) *A Revolution in Social Policy: Quasi-market Reforms in the 1990s*. Bristol: Policy Press Bristol.
Stiglitz J (1990) Principal and agent, in Eatwell J, Milgate M and Newman P (eds) *The New Palgrave: Allocation, Information and Markets*, pp. 241–53. Basingstoke: Macmillan.
Strong N and Waterson M (1987) Principals, agents and information, in Clarke R and McGuinness T (eds) *Economics of the Firm*, pp. 18–41. London: Basil Blackwell.

16 | **Agency in the health sector**

Overview

In this chapter you will explore how the concept of agency operates within the health sector. This will enable you to review the motivational role of incentives in the health sector and the safeguards that need to be applied to ensure the integrity of the agency relationship. You will consider the complexities of agencies in the health sector and revisit the concept of supplier-induced demand (see Chapters 4 and 11) and the complex network of relationships that exist in the provision of health care. This will be done from the perspective of agency theory.

Learning objectives

At the end of this chapter you should be able to:

- discuss the major issues raised by principal–agent theories for a health care system
- recognize the tensions and conflicts of interest peculiar to the health sector that arise between agents and principals
- describe why these tensions or conflicts of interest arise in connection with the governance structures that exist in the health sector.

Keywords

Clinical governance A framework to promote quality improvement in service provision.

Control assurance Concept to promote best practice in clinical governance so as to meet organizational objectives, to protect all stakeholders against risk and to assign responsibility.

Agency in the health sector: the doctor–patient relationship

The traditional application of agency theories in the health sector has been concerned with the relationship between doctors and patients. There is, however, a complex web of agencies that exist in health care, just as in other sectors of the economy. It is important to trace out this web of interrelationships in order to develop a coordinated incentive structure that attempts to ensure that all agents are motivated to achieve the objectives of the organization. This is particularly relevant when evaluating or managing the reformed health care services that have emerged in the past two decades.

Activity 16.1

From what you have already learned, what are the characteristics of the agency relationship in the health sector?

Feedback

The characteristics of the agency relationship you should have identified are as follows:

- asymmetry of information
- effort is not easily observable
- output is difficult to measure
- scope for self-interested behaviour – supplier-induced or supplier-reduced demand
- impact of external factors
- differential power.

How does the agency model translate into clinical practice? Gafni *et al.* (1998) have examined two models – the doctor as perfect agent and the informed treatment decision making model. The authors argue that the transfer of information to the patient is easier than eliciting and transferring the patient's preferences to the doctor in each medical encounter. This is supported by the fact that better technology exists to transfer complex medical information to patients. The second model is more in line with the notion of *consumer sovereignty*.

Both models are based on a one-to-one relationship. However, agency in health care is often a double-sided relationship – doctors may be agents both to patients and to third-party purchasers or payers. Or there may be multiple agents: a patient may expect to be cared for by a number of agents with different skills and levels of expertise, such as a surgeon, anaesthetist and team of nurses and physiotherapists. Each agent will be contributing to the patient's care, and it will be important that they are able to work together for that purpose. In these circumstances it would be necessary to explore the interactions between agents as well as the interrelationship between agents and principals. Different expectations among agents and different incentive structures may affect their combined contribution to caring for patients. Finally, narrowing the doctor–patient encounter to one type of decision making model does not reflect the realities of clinical practice.

Agency in purchasing

One of the issues that has not been resolved in many health care systems is the extent to which purchasers of health services are agents of the payers (i.e. consumers, governments or businesses). Acting as principals buying from the providers, the purchasing team needs to be motivated to draw up the most efficacious service specifications and negotiate the best contract. Often in this case it is not a question of the intermediate agents having more information than their managers. The issue is one of motivating agents to get sufficient information to do the job well by consulting the relevant experts and to ensure that they are up to date on good practice. This involves effort. It is also necessary to ensure that they can not only draw up the most suitable contract, estimating its impact on patient care, but also monitor its execution and make adaptations where necessary. This involves competence and resources.

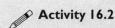 **Activity 16.2**

The following passage from Roberts (1993) discusses the need for government to manage agents' behaviour in the broader context of the managed (or quasi-) markets that were established in the UK in the early 1990s.

As you read it, consider what the main sources of imperfection are in the agency relationships that are central to the UK reforms.

 Managing markets

The purchasing team needs to be motivated to ensure that they draw up the most efficacious service specifications and negotiate the best contract. Yet often the actors in purchasing organizations, even if medically trained, are not expert in all the intricacies of clinical care, and will need to ensure that they have consulted the best authorities and are up to date on methods of good practice. There is rarely the time or the expertise available to do the job well, nor is there much motivation. At present, motivation is based upon professional ethics, performance-related pay and personal career enhancement. There are few penalties for getting it wrong.

There is also some ambiguity in the UK system about who is the principal for whom the agent in the purchasing team is working. Is it the government, the health authority (the purchaser) or the public? How is it proposed that principals, whoever they may be, should discipline purchasers? Having taken away some of the power from professionals, the UK health system is left with purchaser power that is substantial but not well regulated. Purchasers responsible for the health care of the population, and for very large amounts of money, are subject to even fewer disciplines than those that apply to directors in ordinary business enterprises. Performance-related pay, guidelines of good practice and reviews by the various tiers in the health service do not seem adequate.

On the other side, professionals in provider units have to rely upon the managers to negotiate the best terms and secure contracts for their work, and managers in turn have to motivate professionals to perform the work as specified in the contract. To achieve this, budgetary arrangements have been instituted, in the form of resource management, that attempt to make the clinicians financially as well as clinically accountable for their work. These systems are as yet under-developed, and many clinical directors did not have an agreed budget five months into the financial year and few were involved in the contracting process. Both professionals and managers are to be motivated by performance-related pay and monitored by clinical and managerial audit procedures to maintain standards.

The principals will not usually be able to scrutinize the work being carried out or determine the factors that contribute to its success or failure. There are risks involved in any undertaking, and the agents will not always be at fault if health care is ineffective. Systems of controls are needed to ensure as far as possible that organizations bear the responsibility for their failings and do not bear the responsibility for factors outside their control. The design of systems to discriminate in this way is extremely difficult, and excuses for poor performance abound . . . The negotiation of optimal incentive structures, of course, begs the question of whether self-interest does or should propel health care systems.

 Feedback

Factors highlighted include:

- lack of expertise and incentive for purchasers to negotiate best contracts
- ambiguity in the nature of the agency relationships – who is an agent for whom?
- underdeveloped budgetary systems
- difficulties in monitoring performance.

Incentives to reward agents

Those agents working in the NHS in the UK have no property rights in the results of their efforts, except in the case of GP fund holders who, during the period that the fund-holding model was in place, were able to retain some of the surplus and invest it in their practice (Roberts 1998). This lack of potential to share in gains and suffer losses led to some very loose contracting, especially in relation to capital assets.

The drawing up of an incentive scheme to reward agents and ensure that agents execute the work properly is difficult because, in addition to the problems of hidden effort, there is a degree of uncertainty, and external factors may impact on the contract.

Performance-related pay and bonuses have been used to reward higher grades of management. Staff may also be motivated by the possibility of internal promotions – career enhancement and competition with other agents within the organization and in other organizations.

In the UK the introduction of the quasi-market purchaser–provider division appeared to leave the purchasers in much the same hierarchical relationship to central government as had existed before. This may have reflected the inertia that besets organizations during reforms; when individuals and routines remain unchanged the actors may not perceive that they have scope to innovate or adapt their job to take account of the larger structural changes. They may also feel hedged in by constraints on their actions through budgetary stringency (Crawshaw *et al.* 2000).

Should purchasers compete?

Competition from other purchasers may well be a useful discipline, but it is one that is not always available. As agents for consumers, purchasers are in a very protected environment as there is often no accountability to the local population for whom they purchase. And the populations in these areas have few alternative purchasers from which to choose. Introduction of patient choice in this scenario is difficult to implement as purchasers are supposed to be proactive and place contracts where they feel they get the best deal, which is not easy to reconcile with the choices of patients who may wish to be treated elsewhere.

Purchasers face little competition in the UK scheme, unlike the Dutch or German schemes or managed care in the USA where there are often multiple health management organizations (HMOs) or preferred provider organizations (PPOs) from which to choose. The competitive nature of the managed care programmes in the USA is seen in their proliferation and in the items that are stressed in advertisements and promotional literature. Many of these schemes are, in addition, hedged in by a regulatory framework that does not exist to the same extent in other countries which tend to rely more on professional ethics, trust and self-regulation.

In some low income countries the choice is between government health centres, private dispensaries and traditional healers. Heller (1982) examined these options. Consumers in urban areas of low income countries often have a great deal of choice among primary care providers and can also choose among public and private providers and between Western and traditional medicine, if they are able to pay. However, in rural areas the choice is minimal and the availability of services of any kind is sparse.

Agency and providers

The problem of agency is no less evident among health care providers. The negotiation of contracts rarely involves agents who will carry out the work, and the lines of accountability are blurred by the interaction of managerial and professional hierarchies. There is scope for the various agents to behave opportunistically, as there is uncertainty. External factors influence the outcome, and observation of effort is difficult. Unless managers can use the agency relationship to motivate clinicians to perform the work as specified in the contract, they jeopardize the outcome. In these complex relationships, team and cooperative strategies may be more applicable than managerial hierarchies. Incentive structures based on output may well be difficult to establish in health care because of measurement difficulties (of outcomes). Assessors have been used in some health systems to ensure that treatment is as planned and that admissions and discharges occur according to the protocol.

There have been a number of attempts in the reorganized NHS in the UK to harness economic incentives to medical practice. This is illustrated in the introduction of incentives to GPs to achieve certain screening and vaccination targets. GPs receive additional payments when they reach target service levels. Sharing in the property rights of the organization (with the exception of aspects of general practice) is not a feature of the British NHS but has a considerable role to play in some other systems.

Lack of property rights is seen as the factor which some economists believe will prevent internal markets succeeding.

Audit, performance-related pay for managers and financial accountability of clinicians play a part in the management of the agency relationship, as do external factors such as reputation and competitive pressures from peers and other organizations, monitoring schemes and clinical audits, accreditations and so on. These schemes relate to quality improvement and performance management and they can be seen in the context of institutional economics as measures to counteract the problems arising from the agency relationship.

Quality improvement in the British NHS

Recent moves to adopt *clinical governance* as a comprehensive approach to quality improvement in the NHS are a further attempt to gain some leverage over clinical agents. Clinical governance is defined as 'a framework through which NHS organisations are accountable for continuously improving the quality of their services and safeguarding high standards of care by creating an environment in which excellence in clinical care will flourish' (Department of Health 1999).

Accompanying quality improvement is a system of control assurance, defined as

> a holistic concept based on best governance practice. It is a process designed to provide evidence that NHS organisations are doing their 'reasonable best' to manage, direct and control themselves so as to meet their objectives and protect employees, patients, the public and stakeholders against risks of all kinds. This process is complementary to, and proceeds in tandem with, developments in clinical governance and risk pooling in the NHS. (National Health Service Executive 1999)

It remains a problem both for the public and purchasers to obtain accurate information on service quality. In the previous chapter you saw that with asymmetry of information agents tend to 'signal' information on their true type to their principals. The signalling model is reflected in health care as providers under competition tend to communicate information on quality such as the qualifications of their staff and the state of the art of the technologies available to their patients (Robinson 1988).

 Activity 16.3

What do you think might be the limitations or weaknesses of the quality improvement activities in your country?

 Feedback

Often providers have only to demonstrate compliance with certain quality procedures rather than specific outcomes of care. The key problem is who should be responsible and what should be measured? The parameters should allow a meaningful comparison across providers and should take account of differences in case mix. However, quality signals may not reach all who could make use of them and information needs may differ between consumers and purchasers. It is vital to achieve staff commitment to support schemes rather than impose them as external measures.

Self-interest in heath care

Self-interested behaviour, as a key motive in the agency relationship, is expected to be replaced to some extent by the internalized values of professional ethics which ensure that the agent works in the patients' best interests. Group pressures and internal conventions can act in powerful ways to ensure compliance. But group loyalty can also act against the interests of patients.

For example, in a case in Bristol in the UK, two doctors who had carried out substandard heart surgery on young children over a number of years had continued to practise despite colleagues' warnings about their competence (Dyer 1999). This and similar cases of malpractice suggest that there are limitations to the extent to which peer pressure can be relied upon to maintain quality. Monitoring and regulation are clearly needed to disclose major problems while not demotivating professionals or being capable of being subverted by them.

Trust

Trust is a highly valued attribute of relationships among agents and principals and one which is fragile. It can enhance efficiency by cutting down on monitoring costs and allowing scope for agents to operate in a way that they think best given their basic knowledge. Once lost, trust cannot easily be re-established.

Self-interest and altruism are features motivating health care practitioners, and attempts to change the balance towards self-interest may, given the utility functions of clinicians and carers, be counterproductive. In the end, people's internal values determine what they do.

Summary

You have learned about agency in the health sector and looked at agency in doctor–patient relationships. You have learned about the complex interrelationships between individuals and organizations. You have also addressed aspects of agency in purchasing and provision and looked at the role of quality improvement to control the agent. Aspects of agent behaviour, self-interest and trust have also been addressed.

References

Crawshaw SC, Allen P and Roberts JA (2000) Managing the risk of infectious disease: the context of organisational accountability. *Health, Risk and Society* 2(2): 125–41.

Department of Health (1999) *Clinical Governance in the New NHS*, Health Service Circular 1999/065. London: Department of Health.

Dyer C (1999) Bristol inquiry reveals that inspections were inadequate. *British Medical Journal* 318: 1719.

Gafni A, Charles C and Whelan T (1998) The physician–patient encounter: the physician as a perfect agent for the patient *versus* the informed treatment decision-making model. *Social Science & Medicine* 47: 347–54.

Heller PS (1982) A model for the demand for medical and health services in Peninsular Malaysia. *Social Science & Medicine* 16: 267–84.

National Health Service Executive (1999) *Governance in the New NHS: Background Information and Guidance on the Development and Implementation of Controls Assurance for 1999/2000*, Annex A. Leeds: NHS.

Roberts JA (1993) Managing markets. *Journal of Public Health Medicine* 15(4): 305–10.

Roberts JA (1998) *Agathatopia*. Public Health Policy Departmental Publication, London School of Hygiene & Tropical Medicine.

Robinson JC (1988) Hospital quality competition and the economics of imperfect information. *The Millbank Quarterly* 66(3): 465–81.

SECTION 5

Equity in health care

17 | Equity in health care – general concepts

Overview

Much of the book thus far has focused on the role of economics in informing how health systems can be made more efficient, how services can be provided more cost-effectively and how production can be made technically efficient. These are no doubt important and generally reflect the focus of most health economics. Nonetheless, equity is of great importance in the minds of policy makers and citizens in many countries. In this chapter you will examine the concept of equity and the role it plays in the planning and financing of health services.

Learning objectives

After completing this chapter you should be able to:

- **explain the efficiency–equity trade-off**
- **distinguish between vertical and horizontal equity**
- **distinguish between procedural and distributive justice.**

Key terms

Distributive justice Equity as seen in terms of the actual distribution of goods.

Equity Fairness, defined in terms of equality of opportunity, provision, use or outcome.

Horizontal equity The equal treatment of individuals or groups in the same circumstances.

Procedural justice Equity as seen in terms of the processes used to arrive at a distribution of goods.

Vertical equity The principle that individuals who are unequal should be treated differently according to their level of need.

What is equity?

This is a term that is often invoked in policy and academic debates and argued about quite vigorously. This may be particularly so when various protagonists put forward a case against a proposal that may adversely affect one group of the population *vis-à-vis* another. The problem with much of the debate surrounding equity, however, is that little attention is usually given to defining what it actually means.

Before getting into the specifics of equity, three general points are worth considering. First, equity is synonymous with fairness. The problem with fairness as a notion, however, is that what is fair or equitable to you may not be fair or equitable to someone else. It is inherently subjective. Therefore, when deciding what is equitable, it needs to be recognized that whose perspective is taken is crucial to the answer that you will get. As a consequence, the legitimacy of any one specific criterion for equity is often judged by how well it accords with the values of the community. Furthermore, the notion of equity is often clouded in practice by individuals' perception of their own interest.

Second, equity is different from equality. As mentioned above, equity is about fairness. Although this often means ensuring the equal sharing of a good, it is not *necessarily* so. In many circumstances, as discussed later, certain objectives imply the unequal distribution of particular goods.

Third, one account of equity consistent with the conventional utilitarian framework is that an individual's concern for another individual or group in the community is purely instrumental (i.e. your concern for my health is based solely on how it impacts on my utility function). This idea has been labelled the 'caring externality', and, although no doubt important, it does not seem to give a complete account of equity. (This was discussed briefly in Chapter 11.) A potentially significant dimension of equity that is missed by this is the context of the community in which it is invoked. It seems to restrict equity to the question of how much benefit you derive from the well-being of the next person. A perspective that takes into account the community dimension might address broader and perhaps more pertinent constitutional questions such as what type of society we want to live in.

 Activity 17.1

The following passage from an address given by Stephen Leeder (2003) discusses the notion of equity and the differences in how it can be interpreted.

While reading it, think about what it is, from your viewpoint, that makes a society equitable. What role do you see for the state in this type of society?

 Equity versus opportunity

In 1988, I attended a workshop of health care service managers sponsored by the King's Fund of London. Participants included such managers and the odd academic from the United Kingdom, the United States, Canada, Australia and New Zealand. We were discussing resource allocation, and frustration mounted during the first 2 days. Ideologically, participants had divided into two teams – the US and the rest.

On the third day, the leader of the US team said, 'The difference between us is that you guys believe in equity and we don't. In the US, people are less interested in making sure everyone gets care than that those who can get it get great care. They accept not getting care *now* if they can see the opportunity to improve their position and succeed, so that, when they get the money, they will be able to buy great care the minute they want it. It is all about opportunity. People in the US want opportunity, not equity. That's what they think is fair.'

It was important that the US delegate said what he did. It cleared the air. It reminded us that not all societies, and not all people within a society, share a common view of what is fair. In the US, fairness means that you will be encouraged to seek personal success without having to worry much about anyone else.

In the UK, Canada, New Zealand and Australia, there is a general interest in the well-being of others. I doubt that Robert Putnam could have written his book *Bowling Alone* about Australia. Putnam's book mourns the loss of social capital, a resource that grows from community trust and participation. Putnam especially laments its replacement with a fierce individualism.

↻ Feedback

These are big questions, and clearly there are no right or wrong answers! There are numerous approaches, each involving at the outset important value judgements as to what is seen as fair. As seen in the above passage, the difference between the USA and other countries is often fundamentally about values.

One viewpoint broadly sees equity in terms of equality of opportunity, while an opposing viewpoint sees it more in terms of equality of outcomes. The former tends to favour a *laissez-faire* approach to government, while the latter tends to be associated with greater levels of state involvement, particularly in the establishment of a welfare state. Other perspectives view the state not in terms of equalizing outcomes but of ensuring the provision of basic minimum services such as health care and education. Whichever perspective you take, it is worth reflecting on what you believe to be the objective of the social policy maker in your ideally 'equitable' society – and, in turn, the type of health sector that belongs in this type of society.

Equity–efficiency trade-off

In economics, equity is often characterized as conflicting with efficiency. In other words, when attempting to achieve a more efficient health care system, there will inevitably be adverse equity implications. Conversely, if equity is being pursued, there is an opportunity cost in terms of lost efficiency. This, in many instances, might be a reasonable conclusion to draw.

For example, in a district there may be a number of primary care clinics each servicing a local population. A proposal to close down some of these clinics and centralize services could be put forward on the basis of the argument that each clinic essentially performs the same task as the others and therefore, by consolidating, use can be made of possible excess capacity. The equity argument against this proposal would be that by consolidating, geographical access to services would be reduced. How, therefore, might this trade-off between equity and efficiency be quantified? Suppose that the current average cost of a consultation is $20 but would fall to $15 with the introduction of the new policy. It could be argued then that the cost of maintaining a more geographically equitable system (current) is $5 per consultation. Of course, there are other factors that need consideration, as some of the possible $5 cost saving might be offset by greater travel costs for patients. Also, there may be overall reductions in the number of consultations as the increase in geographical barriers associated with the proposal may deter some patients from seeking care.

Another example where such trade-offs can occur is in the introduction of user charges for health services. It is argued that imposing such charges can address the problem of moral hazard by minimizing the frivolous use of services but it is also generally acknowledged that such charges may impose heavy burdens on poorer groups and thereby be inequitable.

A slightly different type of trade-off occurs in community health insurance. The problem in this instance is in ensuring the enrolment of poorer groups who are typically at a higher risk. Risk-rated premiums could be unaffordable to this group and thus viewed as inequitable. Cross-subsidies through community-rated premiums, however, could be more equitable but also promote adverse selection and in turn, undermine the sustainability of such programmes.

User charges have been implemented in numerous countries despite criticism of their equity implications. The following piece provides the views of Andrew Creese (1997), a health economist at the World Health Organization who highlights the problems associated with such fees.

📖 User fees increase inequity

If user fees for health care are the solution, what exactly is the problem? Proponents of user fees recommend them in two situations. The first is when health spending in total is low or falling – fees are recommended as a way to mobilize more money for health care than existing sources provide. The second, paradoxically, is when health expenditure is high or rising quickly, when fees are recommended as a way of improving efficiency by moderating demand and containing costs. Opponents of user fees attack them as a political strategy for shifting health care costs from the better off to the poor and the sick, pointing to the trade-off between this method of raising revenue and maintaining access to care based on need rather than ability to pay.

Dramatic differences exist between countries. Levels of and trends in national income and the condition of health systems vary widely among countries, and local context needs to be considered when making comparisons. In many transition economies such as China, Kyrgyzstan, Georgia, and Vietnam formal and informal charging at subsidized (government) health facilities has been used to replace sharply declining public sector funds. In most of the very poor countries of sub-Saharan Africa fees have been raised or introduced, sometimes after years of commitment to free health care, as a way to provide small but sometimes critical supplements to government health spending of less than $5 per capita.

In these extreme situations fees have been a mechanism for finding additional funding. How successful have user fees been in this context? Measured as a percentage of total government health spending, income from user fees remains at less than 5% in most African countries, although it seems to be somewhat higher in Asia and has risen to as much as 36% in China. But, overall, experience with fees as a device for raising revenue in poor and transitional countries is modest.

User fees can be costly to implement, and income based exemptions in particular have widely proved difficult to manage. Some major shifts in access to and use of health services have been recorded in several countries implementing a policy of user fees, with use in rural areas falling by over 50% a year for several years . . . Increases in maternal mortality . . . and in the incidence of communicable diseases such as diphtheria and tuberculosis have been attributed to such policies . . . A contemporary commentator said of Vietnam [that] access to health care increasingly depends on income, and another said of China [that] access to health care is largely based on the patient's ability to pay, and many cannot afford care.

In the industrialized countries the context is one of comparative economic prosperity and stability and, in the main, of relatively well functioning and accessible health systems. Average per capita health spending in countries of the Organisation for Economic Cooperation and Development in 1995 was over $1500. In Western Europe all countries currently have some limited form of user fee policy, most commonly in the form of partial payment for drugs. Total levels of finance generated through fees for publicly subsidized care are difficult to assess but are probably not very different from those reported for African countries. Levels of spending on health care and growth rates differ among this group of countries, with Bismarckian insurance-based systems generally taking a larger share of gross domestic product and having faster growth rates than Beveridge-type national health systems. . . .

In both types of system, but more so in NHS-type systems (Britain, Ireland, Italy, and Spain), overall control of costs has generally been relatively successful, either through mechanisms of financing through a single source with relatively hard budget limits or through ceilings on premium contributions and reform of provider payments; thus the role of user fees is much more as a tool for moderating demand than a source of revenue. As an instrument for controlling costs by managing demand, user fees have had limited success. From several industrialized countries there is evidence that increasing fees does reduce use of health services, though not necessarily service costs. Reduced use of services has sometimes been accompanied by increased intensity in the form of longer or more expensive treat-ment episodes. In the area of cost control, user fees seem to be a relatively weak policy tool because they focus on patients' behaviour rather than that of providers. Not only are providers a more powerful determinant of health care costs, by making decisions on behalf of patients for all but first contact visits, but changes on the supply side in purchasing and provider payment mechanisms have shown themselves to be more powerful ways of influencing providers' behaviour and service costs . . .

And there remains the question of equity. Shifting the financing base in the health sector, even at the margin, can have profound effects on access to services. No country's experience shows this more clearly than China, where some 800 million people lost their health insurance protection during the 1980s, when rural insurance collapsed and fees grew in importance from 24% to 36% of health care finance. User fees shift the financing burden away from population based, risk sharing arrangements – such as funding based on tax or social insurance – and towards payments by individuals and households. The higher the proportion of user payments in the total mix of financing for health, the greater the relative share of the financing burden falling on poor people. Poor people are both sicker and more sensitive to health care prices than wealthier people. A range of policy options other than user fees exists for dealing with situations of both underfinancing and rapid growth in expenditure. As an instrument of health policy, user fees have proved to be blunt and of limited success and to have potentially serious side effects in terms of equity. They should be prescribed only after alternative interventions have been considered.

In response to this paper, a British GP, Johnathan Reggler (1998), argues that user fees might be appropriate in the UK.

The case for user fees

Creese attacks user fees but fails to make a proper case against them in Britain, basing his arguments predominantly on evidence from countries in the second and third worlds. Creese's statements about the disadvantages of user fees may be true for underdeveloped nations, where absolute poverty is common and the main diseases are infections and illnesses associated with real deprivation. The situation in first world nations is different. Both the media and politicians have encouraged what is effectively a disengaging of demand from absolute need, at least as far as primary care is concerned. As a result, demand spirals upwards while real need increases little, if at all. Ham has described the situation in Singapore, where user fees are the key to reducing demand in a first world system. User fees are also used extensively in western European countries to reduce demand.

Creese believes that supporters of user fees are attracted to them because they will simply reduce total demand. For general practitioners in Britain the point is that user fees will not only reduce total demand (which Creese concedes) but also particularly reduce inappropriate demand, allowing general practitioners to provide a better service for their needier patients.

Creese complains that user fees will bring in little extra revenue and that they do not reduce costs overall. But the aim is not to make the NHS cheaper. It is to bring in a bit more money and to encourage more responsible use of the service, thus allowing the NHS to be more effective. Goldsmith has shown that user fees might increase NHS funding by 5%, although his suggested fees are low and he excludes several services which should be included . . . Nevertheless, 5% is better than nothing.

Finally, Creese argues that user fees increase inequity. He cites evidence from the second and third worlds, where fees are levied on the very poor. In Britain, user fees could be combined with a simple exemption system for poor people, linked to benefits for those with low incomes. It is better for all users that there is slightly less than perfect equity in a system that copes with the reasonable demands placed on it, rather than perfect equity in a system overwhelmed by unreasonable demands. In general practice especially, user fees would achieve the necessary balance.

 Activity 17.2

Discuss the rationale and the possibilities for overcoming Creese's concerns about equity, particularly in low income countries.

Feedback

The general rationale for user charges is twofold: first, they act as a means of rationing demand; and second, they are seen as a revenue-raising mechanism, thereby promoting the financial sustainability of health services. Such charges tend to affect the poorest groups most heavily and potentially deter the use of necessary health services. One possibility for addressing this problem is the use of exemptions for certain disadvantaged groups. However, the evidence as to the effectiveness of such policies in practice is mixed.

> Reggler, in the context of the British NHS, argues that user fees can be important in stemming demand and thus reducing unnecessary costs. The danger, however, is that price rationing of this nature leads to less use of *necessary* services as patients are not always well informed about their health care needs.

Horizontal and vertical equity

Equity can be defined as either horizontal or vertical. *Horizontal* equity is the equal treatment of equals. For instance, it implies that those with the same illness or health need would be given the same treatment. *Vertical* equity, however, relates to how differently individuals in different circumstances should be treated; a definition that is often used is 'the unequal but equitable treatment of unequals'. An example of this concept applied outside health care is progressive taxation and the proportionately higher level of tax the rich are supposed to pay. Analytically, as well as in terms of policy implications, vertical equity is less straightforward than horizontal equity because it requires judgements to be made about *how* different care should be for individuals in different circumstances.

 Activity 17.3

The following excerpt from an article by Gavin Mooney (1996) highlights the lack of recognition of issues of vertical equity and then discusses the possibilities for building in such concerns in Aboriginal health in Australia.

While reading, list some examples of policies that entail the application of vertical equity principles in health care.

 Vertical equity

Alan Williams ... made the point that, for health economists, among the important strategic research issues to be confronted in the next decade is how views about equity are to be incorporated into the measurement process. I want to support that statement. Deciding how best to handle considerations of equity is problematical at any level. They are, as I hope to explain, still greater when dealing with Aboriginal health in Australia. Yet there are problems here which are common to other countries where there are substantial differences in health status within a society. One would hope that a greater proportion of health economists' efforts might go in the direction of research on equity in the next decade. The returns are likely to be high as there seems so much remaining to be done. But then I suppose that depends on how health economists – and others – value research on equity.

In this editorial, Aboriginal health in Australia is used to exemplify the issue of vertical equity which is defined as the unequal but equitable treatment of unequals. (Horizontal equity is the equal treatment of equals.)

The paper also stems from a more general concern about the lack of progress that health economists are making with respect to equity considerations in health care, especially but not exclusively vertical equity. As Adam Wagstaff and Eddy van Doorslaer . . . indicate: 'the issue of vertical equity in the delivery of health care rarely gets discussed in the health economics literature'.

With respect to differences in health status between Aborigines and non-Aborigines in Australia, there are many ways of exemplifying these. Age standardized mortality is approximately 300% of the rate for other Australians. Mortality in the age range 30–34 is over 1000% of the rate for other Australians; infant mortality about two and a half times as great. Diarrhoeal diseases are more than 16 times as common, while end stage renal failure is more than 7 times as high and tuberculosis more than 15 times as great and so on and so on. As Bartlett and Legge . . . indicate, if present health patterns remain unchanged Aboriginal boys would have a 45 per cent chance of living to age 65 (compared with 81 per cent for non-Aborigines) and Aboriginal girls would have a 54% chance of living to age 65 (compared with 89 per cent for non-Aboriginal girls) – poor *vis-à-vis* other indigenous populations, and the gap in Australia greater than in other countries.

The evidence is also clear that any deficiencies that may exist in terms of equity with respect to health services are not being 'made up' through other health enhancing services such as housing, education, water, etc. If anything the situation in these areas is still less equitable than in health services *per se* . . .

Against this background of Aborigines and non-Aborigines within the same society having very different health status and very different health care needs, how can we form a judgement of what would be an equitable provision of health care? While there are features of the situation in Australia which are unique to Australia, there are nonetheless issues common to other countries which have indigenous and non-indigenous peoples. There are also features that other societies share where, for other reasons, there are greatly disadvantaged subpopulations who have much poorer health status than the majority of the population.

 Feedback

Policies that involve targeting disadvantaged groups are typically seen as vertical equity initiatives. Examples include exemptions on user fees, resource allocation formulae that target geographical regions with greater needs, and progressive payment scales used in charging social health insurance levies.

Procedural and distributive justice

The discussion thus far has focused exclusively on the issue of distributive justice – determining what is equitable in terms of the distribution of some good. However, an issue that has recently been attracting some attention is the notion of procedural justice – the issue of how decisions are made in relation to the allocation of resources. Amartya Sen (2002) has argued that decisions aimed at achieving distributive justice might fail on procedural equity grounds if they entail some degree of gender discrimination. In a similar vein, Mooney *et al.* (2002) have examined the issue of procedural justice in indigenous health and have argued that procedural concerns such as community consultation are intrinsic to achieving equity.

Summary

Equity is a massive topic and you have only scratched the surface in this chapter by examining general concepts that will set the scene for more detailed analysis in the next chapter. It is a topic that is enriched (or complicated, depending on how you want to look at it!) by its explicit reliance on ethical and moral considerations. It thus overlaps with political and moral philosophy as well as areas such as health policy analysis, epidemiology and political science.

References

Creese A (1997) User fees. They don't reduce costs, and they increase inequity. *British Medical Journal* 315: 202–3.

Leeder SR (2003) Achieving equity in the Australian health care system. *Medical Journal of Australia* 179(9): 475–8.

Mooney G (1996) And now for vertical equity? Some concerns arising from aboriginal health in Australia. *Health Economics* 5: 99–103.

Mooney G, Jan S and Wiseman V (2002) Staking a claim for claims: a case study of resource allocation in Australian Aboriginal health care. *Social Science & Medicine* 54: 1657–67.

Reggler J (1998) User fees would both yield money and encourage more responsible use of NHS. *British Medical Journal* 316: 70.

Sen A (2002) Why health equity? *Health Economics* 11: 659–66.

18 Equity and health care

Overview

This chapter examines some of the more specific equity criteria that have been applied in the health sector. This follows on from the previous chapter which provided a more general outline of how equity can be put forward as a concept.

Learning objectives

After completing this chapter you should be able to:

- outline the various definitions of equity as applied in the health sector
- identify the fundamental reasons why equal access and equal utilization differ as objectives
- outline the different approaches to measuring need.

Key terms

Access How readily an individual is able to use a service.

Capacity to benefit The extent to which an individual is able to derive some benefit from the use of a service.

Horizontal equity

Although it was suggested that horizontal equity is relatively more straightforward than vertical equity, there are major controversies in this area. The problem with establishing a criterion for horizontal equity is determining precisely the dimensions on which the equality between individuals is to be achieved. The most commonly cited horizontal equity criteria are: equal spending for equal need; equal access for equal need; and equal utilization of equal need. Furthermore, the criterion of equal health is often added into the debate, although this could be interpreted more as a vertical equity objective. At first glance, with the exception of equal health, there does not appear to be much difference between these criteria. However, upon closer examination, subtle but significant differences emerge.

Equal spending for equal need

This is perhaps the weakest criterion; it implies that those individuals with the same level of need should be allocated the same amount of health care expenditure. Crucially, it says nothing about the possibility that spending the same amount on different individuals might yield differences in outcomes because of, among other things, differences in the cost of services between groups or regions (although this is addressed if the criterion is amended to 'equal resources for equal need'), differences in the productivity of resources across groups or regions and differences in the capacity of individuals to get healthy from the same treatment. This criterion also says nothing about how much more or less individuals with different levels of need should be treated relative to one another. The most common application of this criterion has been in resource allocation formulae that have been used to varying extents over the years in the UK, Australia and South Africa (NSW Department of Health 1999; McIntyre *et al.* 2002; UK Department of Health 2003). These formulae generally allocate resources to different geographical regions on the basis of some measure of health need – typically standardized mortality ratios (although other variables are sometimes included such as, in the case of Australia, rural/urban, socioeconomic status and proportion of Aborigines (NSW Department of Health 1999).

Equal access for equal need

In operationalizing this criterion, the task of defining 'access' is crucial. It could simply mean that services should be geographically spread so that people with the same level of need have the same distance to travel. However, this is a fairly narrow interpretation. In principle, 'access' can be taken to mean financial as well as geographical access. Furthermore, broader access issues such as language and cultural sensitivity come to the fore when dealing with the provision of services across different cultural and ethnic groups.

Equal utilization of equal need

This requires policy makers to go one step further and ensure not only that those with the same level of need have the same level of access but also that this then translates into the same level of use. Therefore the difference between equal access for equal need and equal use for equal need emerges if individuals have differing preferences for health. In other words, two individuals with the same access to health and with the same level of need will only use services to the same extent if their preferences for health care and health are the same. In selecting between this and the preceding criterion, the question arises as to how far the health sector should go in imposing upon or shaping people's preferences in this way.

Equal health

A feature of this approach is that it incorporates a very explicit concern for vertical equity and also tends to have strong political appeal. It is perhaps the 'strongest' notion of equity of those set out above. The problem with it is in its operationaliza-tion. The first concern is that health is usually determined by factors outside the health sector – not least of which is genetic disposition – and, therefore, it seems incongruous that such an objective should be set for it. The second issue is that given limited resources for health, it is likely that, in order to achieve this, there is a requirement to not only raise the health of those at the bottom but also, unpalatably, lower that of those at the top.

 Activity 18.1

The following passage from an article by Maria Goddard and Peter Smith (2001) examines the extent to which access to services is equitably distributed in the UK. This passage highlights some of the general issues of principle relating to different notions of equity.

As you read it consider the pros and cons of each of the four criteria of equity.

 Equity of access to health services

The concept of equity of access to health care is a central objective of many health care systems and has been an important buttress of the UK National Health Service since its inception in 1948. Yet the concept nevertheless remains somewhat elusive, and research evidence on the nature and magnitude of inequities, although extensive, proves patchy and difficult to interpret. As a result, it is often not straightforward to decide whether inequities in access pose a significant policy problem, and if so, how they might best be tackled. Many governments have made commitments to tackle inequities in access but making this policy operational will be difficult without a clear picture of what is currently known about equity of access to health care services. The purpose of this paper is there-fore to set out a theoretical framework for assessing studies relating to equity of access to health care. The framework is then used to assess recent research evidence on equity of access amongst socioeconomic groups in UK. Although concentrating on the UK experience as an illustration, the paper uses a general analytic framework which is of direct relevance to researchers from other countries seeking to examine equity of access in a wide variety of institutional settings . . .

This paper focuses on equity in the form of equal *access* to health care for people in equal need. It is important to recognize that this is not necessarily the same thing as equality of *treatment* (for equal need) or equality of *health outcome* . . . Equity of access is purely a supply side consideration, in the sense that equal services are made available to patients in equal need. In contrast, variations in treatment arise from the interaction between supply and demand which depend on the preferences, perceptions and prejudices of both patient and health care provider. Variations in health outcome depend on many factors in addition to the receipt of health care.

The concept of equity of access we address is therefore, at least in principle, an objective notion which is independent of ethical judgement. We do not consider here the issue of vertical equity (does access vary appropriately in accordance with variations in need?). The issue of vertical equity is less commonly addressed and gives rise to profound issues of ethical judgement, related, for example, to the extent to which an element of efficiency should be sacrificed in pursuit of a vertical equity goal.

In practice, almost all empirical studies of equity of access, at least in the first instance, consider variations in *treatment* rather than variations in *access*, and exhibit little or no consideration of any theoretical framework for the research. In many circumstances this compromises the usefulness of the results, and we believe that it is imperative that researchers in this area think harder about the theoretical underpinnings to their work . . .

The horizontal principle of equity addressed by this paper is the extent to which there exists equal access for equal need. This begs the questions: what is need? what is access? These questions lead us to consider concepts related to the quality of health care and the utilisation of health care . . .

Need

Unfortunately, as numerous authors have noted, the concept of the need for health care is far from unambiguous . . . For example:

- does it relate to an individual's level of illness or the capacity to benefit from treatment?
- to what extent should non-clinical contributions to need, such as an individual's social circumstances, be considered?
- how is the relevant concept of health status to be measured? In particular, many studies rely on self-reported illness and the predisposition to report illness may vary systematically between groups.
- at what stage should need be measured? For example, two identical individuals may present to the health services with differences in immediate clinical need because previous health care has been less effective for one individual than the other.

. . . In practice, we found that many studies of inequity have paid only scant attention to the concept of need. One of the following assumptions is usually made:

- Levels of need are the same in each group being studied, meaning that no explicit consideration of need is necessary.
- Levels of need are assessed on the basis of a crude measure, such as self-reported morbidity, thereby assuming that there are no systematic variations between groups in the way that the associated question is interpreted or answered.
- Levels of need are assessed on the basis of a biomedical measure of health status, therefore assuming that there is no systematic variation in the way that such measurements are taken and that unmeasured factors (such as social circumstances) are not relevant to need.
- Levels of need are indicated by the characteristics of the area in which individuals live, rather than their own circumstances. This approach leads to potential problems of interpretation, as an effect observed at the area level may not apply at the individual level (and vice versa).
- Need is considered to be a latent variable which cannot be measured directly but is represented by a set of proxy socioeconomic measures, perhaps inferred from statistical analyses of utilisation of the whole sample under scrutiny.
- Levels of need are indicated by the results of some other study, leading to the potential for circularity in argument if that study itself is based on some measure of utilisation.

Clearly each of these alternatives is in some sense deficient and gives rise to the potential for misinterpretation of results. We must nevertheless assume that some acceptable operational concept of need can be developed. This then allows us to envisage a representative individual from each of the population groups of interest *exhibiting some specified level of clinical (and possibly social) circumstances*, which we define as needs. The interest is then in the extent to which access, utilisation, quality and outcome vary according to the population group in which an individual is located.

Access

The next stage is therefore to formulate an operationally useful concept of access. As noted above, this is a supply side issue and indicates the level of service which the health care system offers the individual. The precise formulation of the notion of access is highly contingent on the context within which the analysis is taking place. Thus, in the US, access is often considered to refer merely to whether or not the individual is insured, and nuances such as the level of insurance or the magnitude of co-payments are secondary. In Europe, however, where almost all citizens are in principle insured, access can be quite a subtle concept. It might, at its most general level, refer to the ability to secure a specified range of services, at a specified level of quality, subject to a specified maximum level of personal inconvenience and cost, whilst in possession of a specified level of information.

Unfortunately few, if any, researchers have explicitly articulated all the components of access noted above. Certainly it is often reasonably straightforward to define the range of services under consideration. However, it is important to note that the quality of service is also an intrinsic element of access which might complicate any examination of access . . . Clearly there is enormous potential for quality issues – such as staff attitude, the condition of premises, waiting time, time spent with patients, and clinical outcome – to vary system-atically between population groups. Yet, because of its elusive nature, few studies seriously address the issue of variations in the quality of access.

Many systems of health care are free of user charges. However, there might be con-siderable variations in the personal costs of using services, and although seeking to equalize personal costs of access is infeasible, there must become a point when they become unacceptable . . . Similarly, although a service is available to all individuals, there may be substantial variations in awareness as to its availability and efficacy, perhaps because of language or cultural differences. Again, to the extent that these are amenable to health service remedy, they may constitute legitimate components of access.

In summary, variations in access offered by the supply side might arise for the following reasons:

- *Availability:* certain health care services may not be available to some population groups, or clinicians may have different propensities to offer treatment to patients with identical needs from different population groups.
- *Quality:* the quality of certain services offered to identical patients may vary between population groups.
- *Costs:* the health care services may impose costs (financial or otherwise) which vary between population groups.
- *Information:* the health care services may fail to ensure that the availability of certain services is known with equal clarity by all population groups.

Although various *indicators* of access (such as availability of resources, waiting time, user charges and other barriers to care) might be measured, it is rarely the case that the complex notion of access described above can be observed directly . . .

Utilisation

The measure of utilisation used may often be problematic. For example, numbers of contacts with a general practitioner may be used as a measure of utilisation in primary care. Yet contact rates may not be a good measure of either the quality or quantity of health care received. Indeed, in some circumstances a contact may simply reflect an administrative requirement, such as the need to obtain a sick note for an employer. Similarly, measures of hospital utilisation such as completed episodes or bed days give rise to problems of interpretation. Many empirical studies focus on utilisation of a single procedure. Yet there may be equally effective alternative health care therapies which are not considered. In these circumstances, underutilisation may simply indicate use of such alternative therapies. Similarly, some groups may make use of alternative services in the private or voluntary sector and thus variations in utilisation of public services will not give a full picture of total use.

We nevertheless assume that a satisfactory measure of utilisation can be found. This allows us to develop an economic model of whether or not an individual receives care, based on the interaction of supply of care (represented by access) and demand for that care. Separating potential influences on utilisation into supply and demand factors provides a useful classification system which allows us to address the important issue of the *causes* of any observed variations. However, we recognize that in many cases supply and demand factors will interact in order to produce observed variations in utilisation for a given level of need, and in such cases it may be difficult to separate them without further analysis.

 Feedback

- Equal health. Pro: has some intuitive appeal since it can be argued that health is the main objective of health care. Con: possibly utopian. It fails to account for the determinants of health that fall outside the remit of the health sector.
- Equal use for equal need. Pro: aims to ensure that those with same health problems have at least the same treatment. Con: fails to account for the possibility that individuals with the same condition may have different preferences regarding health and the use of health services.
- Equal access for equal need. Pro: similar to the previous criterion except it allows for the likelihood that individuals have such differing preferences. Con: such preferences can be seen as the product of an individual's environment and therefore there is an argument for overriding them.
- Equal spending for equal need. Pro: relatively more straightforward to implement from the policy maker's point of view. Con: it is relatively weak. It does not account for differentials in cost, productivity of resources or the propensity of individuals to derive health benefit from treatment.

What do we mean by need?

Underlying each of the horizontal equity criteria above is the concept of need. As discussed earlier, there are various ways in which need can be defined. These include variables such as standardized mortality ratios, socioeconomic status and rurality. In a series of recent, high-profile cross-country comparison studies of equity, measures of self-reported health were used to measure need. These were based on data from national household surveys (Wagstaff and van Doorslaer 2000).

Another definition of need is 'capacity to benefit' (Culyer 1995). This means that individuals are only seen to need a service to the extent to which they can benefit from treatment. The implication is that individual A, who is very sick with an untreatable disease, would be deemed to have less need than individual B, who may be moderately ill but with an ailment that does respond to treatment. As a consequence, if it is decided that more resources should be allocated to those populations with greater need (based on capacity to benefit), then relying only on existing health status measures such as standardized mortality ratios may not be appropriate.

Need or 'basic need' has also been defined as a set of basic goods and services required for sustenance of human life. Health care is often (although not always) identified as a basic need along with goods such as shelter, clean water and food. A basic needs approach to policy making tends to view such goods in terms of individual rights and the objective of public policy to first and foremost address these basic needs across individuals – as reflected, say, in the Universal Declaration of Human Rights of 1948 (see http://www.un.org/Overview/rights.html). Such rights-based approaches, however, can be criticized from an economic perspective because they do not recognize potential trade-offs between such goods, the preferences of individuals and the possibility that the nature of what could be seen as an individual's basic needs will differ according to social context.

The following extract from Culyer (1995) elucidates what this notion of need would mean from an economic perspective.

 Need

If 'need' is to be a practical idea, useful in particular in helping people to allocate health care resources more efficiently and equitably, it has to have particular characteristics, the absence of any one of which makes it virtually useless. Unfortunately, in the common contexts in which the term has been taken seriously (political slogan-mongering and – on quite a different plane – philosophical discourse) at least one of these necessary conditions is always absent. The conditions proposed are these:

1　that its value-content be up-front and easily interpretable;
2　that it be directly derived from the objective(s) of the health care system;
3　that it be capable of empirical application in issues of horizontal and vertical distribution;
4　that it should be service- and person-specific;
5　that it should enable a straightforward link to be made to resources;
6　that it should not, if acted upon as a distributional principle, produce manifestly inequitable results.

Even when each of these conditions is met, 'need' turns out to be at best an incomplete criterion for choosing between different distributions of resources *on grounds of equity*. This seems odd, as nearly everyone thinks of 'need' as something closely bound up with equity (compared, say, with efficiency).

That 'need' is value-laden should be self-evident. The values embodied in various usages are, however, all too often obscure. The difficulty is understandable, for nearly every usage implies both a factual or positive statement (such as 'if person A does not receive entity X, then person A will have demonstrably different characteristics') and a value-laden or normative statement (such as 'if the need is met, the demonstrably different characteristics are better than those if it is not met'). Recognizing that these two aspects are inherent in the idea of 'need' is the first step towards creating a workable concept. 'Demonstrably' is added on the grounds that changes in people's characteristics that are not observable (or that could not become observable through the creation of appropriate instruments to make them so) are not interesting factual statements.

While anyone is free to inject their own values into an idea of 'need', embodying what seem to be the driving values of health services (which will doubtless differ from culture to culture) seems a better way forward if the aim is to create a workable concept that people can actually use (people who, for example, are contractually committed as managers or health professionals to deliver on goals set for them by the system in which they are employed). This turns needs-talk away from *advocacy* (where the writer is essentially urging his or her own values) into *consultancy* (where the writer accepts what are perceived to be the values of his or her clients).

Horizontal equity means treating the same those who are the same in a relevant respect (such as having the same 'need'). Vertical equity means treating differently those who are different in relevant respects (such as having different 'need'). Neither type of equity is operational if the concept of 'need' is not sufficiently quantifiable for judgments of sameness or difference to be made with acceptable precision for the purposes in hand.

For service- and person-specificity one must add prepositions: something (like a specific medical act) has to be 'needed' (is necessary) for something else to be accomplished. We must ask also *for what* it is 'needed' (necessary). And we must also ask *for whom* it is 'needed' (necessary). The first requirement is crucial in health care, for it directs attention towards the crucial question of whether *in fact* (or whether it is *probable that*) the act in question will have the effects (for the better) expected. Since so much in medical (and health) care is of unknown effectiveness (or is even of known ineffectiveness), directing attention in this way alerts one to the possibility that someone may even be seriously ill without there being any reasonable prospect (reasonable in the eyes of those who have examined the matter via, say, randomized controlled trials, overviews or meta-analyses) of medical care effectively changing their characteristics for the better. In such cases, whatever else they 'need', they do not 'need' the sort of health or medical services that might be available. Too many unsubstantiated assertions of 'need' *assume*, rather than *enquire* whether, the acts in question really are *necessary*.

One should *ask for what* it is 'needed' because there ought to be some more ultimate good from which the 'need' in question derives its moral force (for example, health is 'needed' in order that one may 'flourish'). It should be person-specific or, at the planning and management level, group-specific since one must be able to identify who it is that 'needs' whatever is asserted to be 'needed'. One can trivialize these requirements. The statement 'surgeons need manual dexterity' is hardly elucidated by asking 'why?', for the answer may be that 'surgeons need manual dexterity in order to be surgeons'. Nor is the statement 'I need open-heart surgery' much elucidated by the justification 'if I am to live'. However, the statement 'I need prophylactic lignocaine following my heart attack' may be false if I fear the risk of early mortality more than I value the prevention of arrhythmias. And the statement 'I need gastric freezing for my ulcer' is plain false, for gastric freezing will do me no good at all and may do me harm.

The link to resources is there as a necessary condition on the ground that the context in which we most urgently need a workable concept of 'need' is to resolve (or at least inform) questions of resource distribution. While the logic in a statement like 'A needs to be healthy if she is to flourish' might meet the first two requirements, it may fail the third and fourth. One can grant a 'need' for health without granting a 'need' for medical care. A particular ground for denying the second 'need' might be because all known medical care is also known to be ineffective in the case in point. There may be other derivative 'needs' arising from the first claim (such as need for palliative care, or for more research into effective medicine) but, in the state of knowledge as it is, today, these 'needs' may coexist with the absence of 'need' for medical care.

One may as well go further: in many cases it may be possible to argue that there is more than one way of meeting a 'need'. Which one, then, is *really* 'needed'? The answer to this is that it is the one that is most cost-effective. A procedure that is less cost-effective than another cannot be held to be more needed. And even if one is to think of it as equally needed, we may as well try to be *efficient* in the way we meet 'needs' and so commit ourselves to the idea that the procedures that may be 'needed' are those that are the most cost-effective at meeting the 'need' in question. If there should turn out to be more than one of these, then we shall be indifferent between them (if there are no other grounds for preferring one to the other). The 'need' might be met equally well through either means.

One idea of 'need' that nearly meets the requirements laid down is that of capacity to benefit. Its value content can be made clear by elucidating the idea of 'benefit'. If an objective of the health care system is to increase 'health gain' (as it is in Britain), then interpreting 'benefit' in terms of some acceptable measure of health gives the definition the contextual relevance insisted on by the second requirement. If health gain is sufficiently quantifiable for one to be able to identify potential gains as 'more', 'less' or 'same', then the third requirement is met. Moreover, the concept distinguishes between ill health (which may or may not imply a 'need' for health) and a 'need' for medical care (when medical care really is necessary). However, it falls at the fourth hurdle (and also would fail the fifth). If one can identify both the procedures that would (with a sufficient probability of success) generate the benefit and the sorts of patients (actual or potential) who will (probably) benefit, then that is fine, but the idea of 'need' is now becoming subtly transformed from capacity to benefit to a 'need' *for* person- and service-specific resources. This may seem a trivial distinction, but it can easily be shown to have major consequences for resource distributions especially if one is seeking equity in distribution, as will shortly be seen.

A much better definition is this: a need for health care is the minimum amount of resources required *to exhaust a person's capacity to benefit*. This definition has all the good elements of the capacity to benefit notion. It also quantifies the resources that are needed (the inverted commas now being dropped) and hence meets the fourth and fifth requirements. At the planning and managerial level, it may for most purposes be adequate (at least in the National Health Service) to treat capacity to benefit as potential health gain. At more personal levels of application (which would have to be fed into more macro decision-making) the idea of capacity to benefit will often have to take account of more complex dimensions of benefit. For example, my need for surgery for my cancer of the larynx may be inadequately assessed in terms of, say, the probability that I shall live longer having the surgery rather than having irradiation alone. But I may say that I need irradiation rather than surgery on the grounds that I prefer the probability of a shorter life with a more usable voice than a longer life without one. Since some patients undoubtedly do prefer this, the planning and management system should provide for sufficient flexibility to allow me to exercise my choice (assuming, of course, that the values embodied in the health care system include sufficient weight on individual preferences of this sort), hence the importance of feedback into macro decision-making about resource distributions.

It is immediately apparent that all needs do not have to be met. The purpose of the concept is, indeed, to enable people to choose on grounds of equity how resources ought to be distributed *given that there are not enough to go round to meet all needs*. Moreover, since there are needs for things that are not health services, so to distribute resources to health care as to eliminate all need for it would be inefficient (leaving lots of more important needs, even of the same people, unmet elsewhere) and inequitable (one would be meeting the trivial needs of those needing health care while leaving those of people needing other things unaddressed and one may even be worsening the distribution of the unmet needs too).

 Activity 18.2

What is the relationship between the notions of capacity to benefit and cost-effectiveness?

 Feedback

Both are seen as criteria on which to allocate health sector resources. Capacity to benefit tends to be invoked in discussions about equity, while cost-effectiveness arises when discussing efficiency. However, in principle, they are effectively the same if the measure of benefit used under capacity to benefit is the same as the measure of health gain used to determine cost-effectiveness. For example, if benefit is defined as reduction in mortality and effectiveness defined as lives saved, then the two principles should result in the same patterns of resource allocation. Both, in this instance, would involve allocating resources to where the greatest marginal gain can be achieved in terms of lives saved. Thus a criticism that could be levelled at the principle of allocating according to need as defined by capacity to benefit is that it may be no different from allocating resources on conventional efficiency grounds.

How do we decide between objectives?

So how do you decide between the competing notions of equity outlined in this chapter? One possibility may be to ask the community. The other may be to examine existing policy documents. In relation to the latter, Donaldson *et al.* (2004) find that in the UK there is some support for the objective of equal access for equal need; in the USA, no explicit equity objective; and in Canada, equal use.

Summary

You have learned about the various definitions of equity that have been discussed in relation to health care. These were: equal health; equal use for equal need; equal access for equal need; and equal spending for equal need. You have also examined more closely the notion of 'need' and, in particular, the implications of defining it in terms of capacity to benefit.

References

Culyer A (1995) Need: the idea won't do – but we still need it. *Social Science & Medicine* 40: 727–30.

Donaldson C, Gerard K, Jan S, Mitton C and Wiseman V (2004) *The Economics of Health Care Financing. The Visible Hand* (2nd edn). London: Macmillan.

McIntyre D, Muirhead D and Gilson L (2002) Geographic patterns of deprivation in South Africa: informing health equity analyses and public resource allocation strategies. *Health Policy* 17 (Suppl.): 30–9.

NSW Department of Health (1999) *Resource Distribution Formula. Technical Paper, 1998–99 Revision.* Sydney: NSW Department of Health.

Goddard M and Smith P (2001) Equity of access to health care services: theory and evidence from the UK. *Social Science & Medicine* 53: 1149–62.

UK Department of Health (2003) *Resource Allocation: Weighted Capitation Formula.* London: Department of Health.

Wagstaff A and van Doorslaer E (2000) Equity in health care financing and delivery, in Culyer AJ and Newhouse JP (eds) *Handbook of Health Economics*, Vol. 1B. Amsterdam: North-Holland.

Glossary

Access How readily an individual is able to use a service.

Accounting approach An approach that uses accounting information (e.g. financial reports) as the basis for undertaking a costing exercise.

Adverse selection When a party enters into an agreement in which they can use their own private information to the disadvantage of another party.

Agency relationship The relationship that exists between trading parties when one (the agent) works on behalf of another (the principal).

Agent A person who acts on behalf of another (the principal).

Allocative (Pareto, social) efficiency A situation in which it is not possible to improve the welfare of one person in an economy without making someone else worse off.

Asset specificity Characteristics of assets that determine whether they are redeployable or not. There are four types of asset specificity: site, physical asset, human asset, and dedicated asset.

Average cost Total costs divided by quantity.

Bliss A transaction in which parties engage to their mutual advantage using a classical contract.

Bounded rationality Behaviour that is intendedly rational, but only limitedly so. There are limits of knowledge and capacity that compromise efforts to behave rationally.

Capacity to benefit The extent to which an individual is able to derive some benefit from the use of a service.

Capture (self-interest) theory This regards regulation as being supplied in response to the demand of interest groups.

Cardinal utility When the utility of individuals can be measured numerically and thus a score of, say, 2 represents twice the value of a score of 1. Cardinality is an important requirement for the aggregation of individual utilities.

Clinical governance A framework to promote quality improvement in service provision.

Consequentialism The notion that it is only the end states that matter – in other words, the ends will justify the means. Utilitarianism, with its emphasis on individual utility, is generally seen as consequentialist.

Constant returns to scale Situation existing when a proportionate increase in all inputs yields an equal proportionate increase in output.

Consumerism The readiness of consumers of health care services (patients) to exercise their choices in markets, actively seeking out and comparing information on price and quality.

Contestable market A market where monopolistic behaviour is disciplined by the threat of entry into the market by other firms.

Control assurance Concept to promote best practice in clinical governance so as to meet organizational objectives, to protect all stakeholders against risk and to assign responsibility.

Cost function The relationship between outputs from production and total costs.

Demand function The relationship between quantity demanded and all other influencing variables.

Derived demand Demand for an item not for its own sake but for use in the production of goods and services.

Diminishing returns to scale Situation existing when a proportionate increase in all inputs yields a less than proportionate increase in output.

Distributive justice Equity as seen in terms of the actual distribution of goods.

Economies of scope Situation where it is possible to produce two or more different products together more cheaply than would be the case if they were produced separately.

Equilibrium A state where (in the context of the market) supply is equal to demand and price is stable.

Equity Fairness, defined in terms of equality of opportunity, provision, use or outcome.

Externalities Costs or benefits arising from an individual's production or consumption decision which indirectly affects the well-being of others.

Extra-welfarism An alternative to utilitarianism in which an objective other than utility is posed as a social goal, often defined in terms of health gain or health-related utility.

Financial (budgetary) cost The accounting cost of a good or service usually representing the original (historical) amount paid – distinct from opportunity cost.

Fixed cost A cost of production that does not vary with the level of output.

Giffen good A good with a positively sloped demand curve – as the price falls, less is demanded.

Governance The means by which order is accomplished in a relation in which potential conflict threatens to undo or upset opportunities to realize mutual gains.

Government failure When the objective of public policy action is undermined by the diverging interests of decision makers within government.

Hirschman–Herfindahl Index A measure of the degree of market concentration, aimed at estimating the competitiveness of the market, and defined as the sum of squared market shares of all firms in the industry.

Homogeneous goods Goods which seem identical in the eyes of the consumer.

Horizontal equity The equal treatment of individuals or groups in the same circumstances.

Horizontal integration (of production) Union or merger of firms at the same stage of production.

Human capital approach An approach that uses wages to measure the value of productivity lost through illness.

Impacted information When information resides with the agent it may be impacted; there would be high costs to achieving information parity.

Income effect The effect of a change in real income on quantity demanded, when relative prices are held constant.

Increasing returns to scale Situation existing when a proportionate increase in all inputs yields a more than proportionate increase in output.

Incremental unit cost The change in costs associated with an increase or decrease of input by an increment (may be several units) that makes sense managerially.

Indifference curve A curve which shows all combinations of commodities that yield the same amount of utility to the consumer.

Informational asymmetry A principal recognizes his or her own information deficit and the superiority of the agent's information.

Interpersonal comparisons of utility Comparisons of measures of utility across individuals, that is, involving judgements of whether individual A gains more (or less) utility than person B from the consumption of a good.

Isocost A line which shows all combinations of inputs that represent the same total cost to a firm.

Isoquant A line joining up all combinations of inputs that produce the same quantity. The convex portion of the line indicates the technologically efficient combination of inputs.

Laissez faire Economic philosophy that relies on market mechanisms to allocate goods and services.

Long run Time period when all factors of production can be varied.

Managerial utility function A function that states that managerial utility is determined by salary, security, power and status.

Marginal cost The change in the total cost if one additional unit of output is produced.

Marginal rate of substitution The rate at which a person will give up one unit of a particular good or service in order to get more of another good or service while deriving the same level of utility (remaining on the same indifference curve).

Marginal rate of transformation The slope of the production possibility curve, indicating the degree of substitutability of one input for another in the production process.

Marginal revenue The change in total revenue resulting from selling one more unit of output.

Market failure The failure of an unregulated market to achieve an efficient allocation of resources.

Maximand (objective function) A particular variable whose maximization is seen to be a relevant social goal. For instance, utilitarians pose utility as the maximand, whilst extra-welfarists might pose health gain.

Monopolistic competition A market model which combines elements of monopoly (a downward-sloping demand curve) with competition (many sellers).

Monopoly Situation where there is only one supplier of a product.

Monopsony Situation where there is only one buyer in the market.

Moral hazard Situation in which one of the parties to an agreement has an incentive, after the agreement is made, to act in a manner that brings additional benefits to themselves at the expense of the other party.

***n*-firm concentration ratio** A measure of the degree of market concentration, aimed at estimating the competitiveness of the market, and defined as the aggregate market share of the *n* largest firms in the industry.

Normal profit The rate of return that is earned in a competitive market. It is usually incorporated in costs. If profits above normal are earned the market will attract new entrants unless there are barriers to entry.

Normative economics Economic statements that prescribe how things should be.

Oligopoly A market that contains only a few firms.

Operational (technical, productive) efficiency Using only the minimum necessary resources to finance, purchase and deliver a particular activity or set of activities (ie avoiding waste).

Opportunism Situation where one party involved in a contract acts in his or her self-interest at the expense of the other party.

Opportunity (economic) cost The value of the next best alternative forgone as a result of the decision made.

Ordinal utility Accepts that utility states can only be ranked as opposed to being measured cardinally.

Positive economics Economic statements that describe how things are.

Potential Pareto improvement (Kaldor–Hicks principle) The basis for cost–benefit analysis. It stipulates that a reallocation of resources which makes someone better off and someone worse off represents an improvement only as long as those who gain could *potentially* compensate those who lose.

Principal A person on whose behalf an agent acts.

Prisoners' dilemma or collective action problem Situation where the collective interests of a group are inconsistent with the individual interests of its members. The problem with achieving the necessary cooperation amongst group members is that, in cooperating, each individual opens him- or herself to exploitation from the others.

Procedural justice Equity as seen in terms of the processes used to arrive at a distribution of goods.

Procedural rationality Where agents do not necessarily succeed in maximizing their own goals but give each decision deliberation that is appropriate to its relative importance.

Production function The functional relationship that indicates how inputs are transformed into outputs in the most efficient way.

Public choice theory This sees government action as a product of the interaction between voters, politicians and bureaucrats.

Public good A Good or service that can be consumed simultaneously by everyone and from which no one can be excluded.

Public interest approach In contrast to public choice theory, this approach sees government action as the necessary means of addressing market failures and/or the inability of markets to achieve certain social objectives.

Purchaser-driven competition Market models in which the drive to shop around for superior price–quality combinations is dominated by institutional purchasers (health maintenance organizations or insurers)

Rationality A key assumption of the utilitarian framework. It sees individuals as being motivated solely by self-interested utility maximization.

Reputation goods Goods in which quality can only be judged by consumers through experience.

Revenue maximization Maximizing the amount the firm earns by selling goods or services in a given period of time – this is different from profits, which are the excess of revenues over costs.

Risk selection The behaviour of insurers or providers who try to avoid patients with higher than average risk of illness.

Shadow price A value which has been adjusted to reflect the opportunity cost of a good or service.

Shadow pricing Prices derived from values expressed elsewhere in the economy.

Short run Time period when at least one factor of production cannot be varied.

Statistical approach An approach in which an econometric model is built to give an idea of how total costs change in response to differences in service mix, inputs, input prices and the level of output.

Substantive rationality Where rational agents maximize the achievement of their own goals, given existing constraints.

Substitution effect The change in quantity demanded of a good resulting from a change in the commodity's relative price, eliminating the effect of the price change on real income.

Sunk costs Costs that are non-recoverable.

Supplier-induced demand Increased demand as a result of a provider (e.g. a doctor) exploiting an asymmetry of information.

Supranormal profits Profits earned by a natural monopolist not threatened by new entrants.

Target income Part of the supplier-induced demand model which postulates that demand inducement is geared to the achievement of some target level of income.

Theory of the second best Theory providing the economic rationale for government intervention in situations of market failure.

Transfer payments Payments which are made between parties without any expected returns to current output or production – for example, social security payments.

Uncertainty Situation in which it is not possible to know or even predict the likelihood of an event occurring. This notion is distinguished from that of 'risk', where probabilities are known.

Utilitarianism (welfarism) Based on the notion that society's interests are best served through the maximization of individual utilities.

Variable cost A cost of production that varies directly with the level of output.

Vertical equity The principle that individuals who are unequal should be treated differently according to their level of need.

Vertical integration (of production) Union or merger of firms at different stages of production.

Welfare economics The branch of economic theory that addresses normative questions.

Index

Page numbers in *italics* refer to tables, figures, 'Activities', and 'Feedback'.